Working with
Dysfluent Children

Working with

Dysfluent Children

Practical Approaches to Assessment and Therapy

Revised Edition

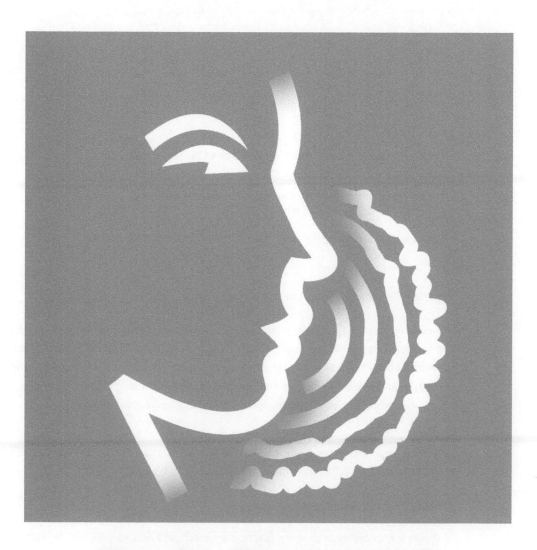

Trudy Stewart & Jackie Turnbull

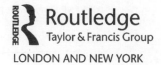

Routledge
Taylor & Francis Group

LONDON AND NEW YORK

DEDICATION

This book is dedicated to those dysfluent children and their families who have taught us so much, and to our own children and partners who have encouraged and supported us in our work.

Note: For the sake of clarity alone, this text uses 'he' to refer to the client and 'she' to refer to the clinician.

First published 2007 by Speechmark Publishing Ltd.

Published 2017 by Routledge
2 Park Square, Milton Park, Abingdon, Oxon OX14 4RN
711 Third Avenue, New York, NY 10017, USA

Routledge is an imprint of the Taylor & Francis Group, an informa business

British Library Cataloguing in Publication Data
Stewart, Trudy
    Working with dysfluent children: practical approaches to assessment and therapy – 2nd rev. ed. –
    (A Speechmark practical therapy manual)
    1. Speech disorders in children 2. Speech therapy for children
    I. Title II. Turnbull, Jackie
    618.9'2855

    ISBN-13: 9780863885143 (pbk)

Printed and bound by CPI Group (UK) Ltd, Croydon, CR0 4YY

Contents

TABLES

FIGURES

Handouts

Foreword

A new edition needs to build on the strengths of the earlier work. With this in mind, I have taken the liberty of retaining the final paragraph of the foreword written by C. Woodruff Starkweather to the 1995 edition of this book. He refers to therapy as a special conversation between equal participants but with different perspectives.

> They sail together in waters that are only partially charted. Each has a map, but the two maps are very different. Clients know their own problem in painful detail; their map is very detailed but covers only a small area. Clinicians know the problem more broadly having studied the literature and been influenced by clients: their map covers a much wider area, but it is missing many details. Together they navigate their way, sharing their different kinds of information. Both end up in a new, sometimes unanticipated, place. My wish for those who use this book, both clients and clinicians, is that they find in their new land the delights of speaking freely.

We can push the sailing analogy further; we can view being a therapist as a long journey of discovery and work with individual clients as shorter trips along the way. During this long journey, professional and personal developments rub shoulders. If we are fortunate, clients, colleagues, personal study and research guide and inspire us and so the therapy we offer becomes more effective. This book gives insights into the journeys made by Stewart and Turnbull and so we benefit from the discoveries they have made.

Two of their important discoveries were Kelly's Personal Construct Psychology and Starkweather's Demands and Capacities Model. Over the years, they have developed their own model, a version of DCM that places a greater emphasis upon personal meanings. The authors have been committed to furthering their own understanding of stammering and therapy and so draw on a wide literature to illustrate and support their approach to therapy. However, they are also pragmatists, they want to get the job done and so they illustrate the therapy concepts with practical guidelines, lists and suggested programmes of work.

The reader may choose to go on a journey with this book; there are things to think about, to admire, to question, to disagree with and to smile about. The book invites the reader to consider their knowledge and beliefs about stammering and how these in turn influence selection of therapeutic methods and activities. Others may prefer to use it as a resource, selecting just the parts pertinent to their particular current enquiry with maybe young children, children in middle years or young adults in secondary school. Either way there is plenty within this book to guide therapists on their journeys with young clients.

Rosemarie Hayhow
Stammering Specialist SLT
United Bristol Healthcare (NHS) Trust
Speech and Language Therapy Research Unit
Frenchay Hospital
Bristol

Preface

The aim of this book is to analyse the practical experiences of dysfluency in children, to look at the ways of approaching those difficulties in collaboration with the child, parents and carers, and to share ideas about therapy techniques which we have found useful. To fulfil those aims it is necessary to outline some of the theory currently underpinning clinical management of non-fluent children and to examine some of the principles upon which intervention is based. However, as with other titles in this series, the focus of the book will be on practical aspects of the problem, with case studies, suggestions, and ideas for therapy at each stage.

OUR STARTING POINT has to be the child. The door to our clinic opens; perhaps it is a three-year-old who walks in, clinging to the leg of his parent, or maybe it is a confident-looking teenager wearing his designer t-shirt and the latest fashion in trainers. Separated by age and appearance, they share a common problem – they have been identified as having dysfluent, or stammering speech. Each individual child or carer with whom we come face to face asks in his or her own way what help the clinician can provide. We ask ourselves the same question, but in answering it we are always aware of how little we really know about the nature, cause and treatment of non-fluency in children of all ages. With these anxieties in our minds, we greet our clients.

DEFINING STAMMERING

Many people have attempted to define the nature and characteristics of stammering, almost for as long as the problem has been recognised. Twenty-first century definitions range from those concerned with ætiology to those that attempt comprehensively to describe stammering in terms of behaviours. While there are as many definitions as there have been researchers, most refer specifically to stammering in adults. These 'adult' definitions reflect a more fixed set of behaviours, beliefs and experiences, and do not address the issues of transience, varying levels of awareness within the speaker, and the competing developments of, for example, language and fluency that are often part of the difficulties in managing dysfluency in children.

If we were to propose yet another definition of stammering appropriate for dysfluency in children, our definition would include:

◆ A differentiation of fluent from stammering speech
◆ A differentiation of normal non-fluency from stammering
◆ A holistic view of children, their developmental stage and their communication contexts
◆ An applicability across the range of clients presenting for diagnosis, from onset to adulthood
◆ The development of covert features of stammering – emotional, psychological, and/or cognitive issues

- Application and relevance to the simplest set of data, observed and/or recorded speech in any setting
- A reflection of current research and clinical understanding of stammering.

We hope this text will go some way towards addressing these issues.

PRIORITISATION

We have called the opening chapter of this second edition 'starting points'. Having considered in general terms what stammering in children might be about, we would like now to turn our attention to what is very often the starting point of our professional involvement with children and their families. As a clinician, you might consider that your first introduction to a child would be a formal one, for example, a letter from a general practitioner, health visitor or other professional – the referral letter. However, it is our experience that parents, carers and other professionals are now much more aware of services available (or lack of them) and are actively involved in seeking out appropriate help for their needs and those of their children. As a result, we often receive telephone calls from parents/carers and professionals wanting specific information on a treatment technique, a piece of research, or to know what we have to offer in our service. These requests can be difficult to give without knowledge of the child concerned and his particular home circumstances. We have therefore devised a set of criteria that we believe identify children who need detailed investigation and for whom this 'immediate' response is inappropriate. This checklist (shown below, and given in table form [Handout 1] at the end of the chapter) can also be applied to the more formal referral letters we receive as a way of prioritising waiting/initial assessment lists. We recommend that services take into account these issues when prioritising children who stammer. In our experience, development of covert stammering behaviours, including avoidance, fear and anxiety when speaking, and the appearance of tension and struggle in the overt symptoms are of particular concern. We will discuss these aspects in more detail in later chapters.

- Anxiety expressed by the child, parent, other relative, carer or other professional
- Identification of the child as having a problem, including the use of the label 'stammerer'/'stammering'

- Avoidance behaviours, including word substitution, rephrasing and/or not talking, and the development of other covert features of stammering
- Teasing or bullying by peer group because of speech
- Instructions to the child to modify or change speaking in some way; for example, to take a deep breath, slow down or say it again
- Presence of struggle and/or tension in the child during or in anticipation of speech, which may or may not lead to the occurrence of blocks or prolongations during speech
- Feeling by the child that his speech is 'out of control'
- Fear/anxiety associated with speaking (that may be specific to a certain situation) which may be anticipated by or present in the child during the event
- The child's inability to say what he wants to say at the time he wishes to say it
- Changes in the way the child behaves and/or communicates; for example, more aggressively, appearing more withdrawn, speech varying according to the situation
- Family history of stammering.

BASIC PRINCIPLES OF THERAPY

We now turn our attention to three basic principles for speech & language therapists for the management of children who present with dysfluent speech:

- The child in context
- Focus on the individual
- An open, non-judgemental therapeutic approach.

These principles are not solely applicable to non-fluent clients, but in general terms can be seen as universal 'truths' relevant to any client-clinician relationship. They are, however, principles that we apply in our work with this population of young dysfluent children. We will discuss each principle in turn, and detail particular aspects that are relevant for these children.

Clinicians may find these points useful in relation to case-history taking and we have therefore included a summary sheet at the end of this chapter.

THE CHILD IN CONTEXT

In our treatment of non-fluent children, we do not treat the speech symptoms in isolation. While we are interested in the nature of the stammer, how it presents, and how severe and frequent it is, there are also other aspects of the child that are of concern. Speech fluency cannot be isolated from the other developmental processes that are simultaneously taking place in the child. The interaction of these processes may be crucial in the management of a child's difficulties.

In addition, children do not operate in a vacuum, but exist in contexts in which communication often takes place. Management of the communication problem must therefore take into account these contexts, and may require changes in them in order for a child to feel more in control.

The Communication Context

The following are some issues to consider in the communication context in which children try to get their messages across.

Important others

In this category we include all those people who are important in children's lives. For younger children these are most likely to be family members or those acting in loco parentis, but as they grow older, others may take on increasing significance. Not only does the influence of friends become more apparent, but a number of other significant adults may affect a child's developing view of himself. In our discussion below we refer to 'parents' but invite readers to replace this with 'childminder', 'relative', 'teacher', and so on, as appropriate.

What feelings might these important others be experiencing?

Guilt   Many parents feel guilty, although they may or may not be able to express their guilt. From our own and others' experience, we see guilt as almost an intrinsic part of parenthood! We often blame ourselves for all manner of attributes or behaviours in our children, assuming these must be our fault and the results of our own actions or lack of them. If you have a child who is dysfluent, it is not unusual that your guilt may be linked to the occurrence of the dysfluency. This guilt is often reinforced by others ('he never stammers at *our* house'), by the earlier advice of GPs ('just ignore it, it will go away'), and by the probing questions that we, as clinicians, often ask ('how do you react when he stammers?'). It may also be accentuated by information in books or from professionals which may suggest the 'right' way of parenting or of behaving towards dysfluent children, to which we can never aspire. For example, if we read or are told that we should reduce our speech rate with our dysfluent child, but we fail no matter how hard we try, guilt may be inevitable and increase the feeling that 'it's all our fault'.

Blame   Parents may want to apportion blame for a child's dysfluency. Blame is sometimes placed on another person ('his Dad never has any time for him, he's always too busy', 'he was fine until he started playing with a boy in the street who stammers'). It can be placed on an event (jealousy of a new baby, moving house, having an operation). Family history might be seen as the cause ('his Dad and his Granddad both stammer'). Some cultures place more emphasis on physical causes ('it's what he eats', 'it's his tonsils'). Putting blame on an identifiable cause may help in alleviating guilt or can be more helpfully understood as the parents' way of trying to make some sense of the problem.

Anger   Another emotion often felt by parents in relation to problems in their children is anger. 'Why has it happened to my child?' The anger may sometimes be directed at a specific person; for example, the doctor who said the child would 'grow out of it' over a year ago, or Granny who's a bit deaf and can never understand what he is saying and constantly asks for repetitions. It has also been our experience that there are families who can feel quite negative towards intervention/therapy of any sort. Sometimes this is because of previous events, advice they have received and/or negative experiences with practitioners that, in hindsight, they believe to be less than helpful. We need to be sensitive to these emotions in our interactions with carers.

Embarrassment/Shame   Parents sometimes feel embarrassed by their child's dysfluency. They may feel embarrassed for the child in anticipation of others' reactions, real or imagined. The shame may be for themselves: the stammer can seem to invalidate their construing of themselves as good parents, and they may therefore try to prevent others from knowing about it.

Threat   Dysfluency can also be construed as a threat to parental hopes and ambitions for their child, and cause high levels of anxiety. Parents may fear for the future of the child – will schooling be affected, how will they cope with speaking French, will they make friends, get married, get a good job? It seems that, as parents, we have a tendency to worry for our children as if they were older, rather than being able to stay in the here and now. One possible reason why anxiety is often so high in parents of dysfluent children is that stammering is so public. Parents cannot keep it hidden in the family. Different families not only place very different expectations on their children but the overtly expressed message ('I just want him to be happy') may have underlying implications (for example, being happy means getting a good job and earning lots of money). Thus dysfluency can represent a threat to the parents' hopes for their child, either in the short term ('I want him to stick up for himself at playgroup') or in the longer term ('I want him to be good at speaking French'). Perhaps, as a result, pressure maybe put on children to 'try harder' or, conversely, a child is construed as incapable of meeting these expectations.

What attitudes might these 'important others' have about speech?

Attitude to speech   We need to understand how family members construe speech in general and fluency in particular. We find it helpful to get to know their feelings about speech. Do they correct children's sounds and grammar; do they insist on particular responses ('please', 'thank you', 'may I leave the table?')? Is 'correct' speech seen as important? Do parents expect their children to use the 'correct' word ('dog' not 'doggy') or to know the names of colours, animals, and so on, at age two? We may also want to understand how they see stammering. What sort of a problem is it for the family? What does it represent? If they know anyone else who stammers, how is this person viewed? Are they construed as 'painful to listen to', as a family we knew construed a relative who stammered? If so, what are the implications for the child who is dysfluent? If that person has had speech and language therapy, what was the outcome? Do they advise the family or child on what to do? In our experience, it is not uncommon for a relative who stammers to offer advice such as 'use a different word' or, in the case of one of our clients, teach the three-year-old prolonged speech!

Attitude to dysfluent speech We need also to think about the function the dysfluency serves for the family. Perhaps it holds together a troubled family by giving them an alternative focus for their difficulties. Maybe it provides a role for a mother who has little else in her life. Sometimes it can be construed as evidence that a child is just like his parents in some way – for example, like Dad in that he is seen as sensitive, insecure, quiet, unambitious, lazy, and so on. A dysfluent child may become the ally of one family member and a 'problem' for another. Trying to understand and make sense of the meaning that the dysfluency has for any particular family must be seen as an underlying principle of any therapy that we undertake.

We are often aware of a family taboo on mentioning a child's dysfluency. The extent to which this should be openly discussed in families is a complex issue but, surprisingly, one that is discussed little in the literature. In the past, the view was that dysfluency should not be discussed with very young children, even if it was very severe, as mentioning it could make them aware that their speech was different and thus reinforce or worsen the problem. While we would still concur with this view for children who appear to have no awareness of any difficulty in speaking, we would warn against the setting up of a 'conspiracy of silence' in which any mention, however circumspect, is seen as taboo. Let us take the situation of an imaginary four-year-old with some struggle behaviour, occasionally severe, who sometimes seems to cut short his utterances or become quieter than usual. If we are able to show him that we can understand his distress, perhaps by discussing how difficult talking is and how the words sometimes do get stuck, we are reacting to him in the much the same way as we might to any other kind of distress he may have (for example, over a broken toy, an argument with a friend or a cut finger). If, on the other hand, we ignore his distress and pretend nothing is wrong, he may wonder why we have not recognised that he is having some difficulty or even whether perhaps the dysfluency is too bad to mention.

Our experience in working with adults who stammer has confirmed our view that stammering is often not mentioned to children who are obviously aware and concerned about it. Adults have told us that, as a result, it became something they kept inside themselves and tried hard not to show. Starkweather echoed this view when he stated:

If parents pretend that nothing is happening when the child stutters, the child will deny the problem or believe that listeners don't realise it is occurring. If, on the other hand, parents are openly willing to talk about the child's dysfluency, the child will not hesitate to perform it and will show less struggle and avoidance. (1987, p165)

We are aware, however, that we often walk a tightrope in helping a parent to decide whether or not to mention the dysfluency. We know there is a danger in creating a problem for the child where none has previously existed. We bear in mind something expressed to us by an ex-client. He asked our advice as to how he could best help his two-year-old dysfluent daughter. He was unsure of whether he should be intervening in any way and recalled, 'I remember my stammer was not a problem to me until the grown-ups made it one.'

Communication Dynamics Within the Family

If we consider the behaviours of parents towards their dysfluent children, we need always to do so in the context of the meaning of the dynamics within the family. When we consider communication, we think about those involved in the communication and the behaviours taking place that are particularly relevant.

Siblings

We now consider the specific views and reactions of other siblings. Many younger children are totally unaware that their brother's or sister's speech is dysfluent, but it is often very apparent to an older child, who may react to it in a variety of ways. Perhaps they will ask questions: 'Why do you talk funny/take so long to say things/keep saying the same word over and over?'. They might find it frustrating and not be prepared to listen or, conversely, might be over-sympathetic and anticipate the other child's needs, not letting him speak for himself. Jealousy may result if a dysfluent child is given more time and attention or is allowed to break some of the rules – for example, to interrupt. The dysfluency can be used as a handy weapon in any verbal confrontation. Sometimes, these reactions help us make some sense of the meaning of the dysfluency for children. For example, we might understand why a very young child is becoming quieter in the context of an older sibling's negative remarks about his speech. The way in which the family deals with these reactions also helps us understand more about their construing of the problem. For example, if they discipline the older child for making an enquiry, rather than giving him an answer to his question, it may indicate the seriousness with which they view the dysfluency and their perception of it as something not to be mentioned.

Listening

Intuitively, it seems to make sense to most parents that listening to children is important. How else can we really get to know and understand them? Of course, there are also families in which this is not the case. Perhaps parents in such families see their role more in terms of 'telling' their children what to do. Children can be construed as 'being good' when they are quiet. In some homes, the television is on continually, the child is frequently absorbed in Playstation or computer activities, and conversation takes second place. There may be so many people in the household that it is difficult for anyone to say all they want.

Yet, even when listening is perceived as important, it is not as easy as it may sound. Many parents lead very busy lives, and the time they are able to spend with their children is limited. Other activities may get in the way too: the washing has to be done, the meals prepared, the phone answered. There are likely to be other people making demands on the parents' time: their other children, their partner, friends and relatives. When time is available, the child may not want to talk; he may be involved in something else, or it may just be the wrong time. Listening to a dysfluent child can be even more difficult. For a start, it takes more time. Parents may think they know what the child is taking so long to tell them. It can be hard to concentrate on *what* the child is saying when parents are so aware of *how* he is saying it. They may want to 'put it right' rather than listening passively and letting the child continue.

We will consider difficulties in listening in more detail later in this book, and specifically in terms of 'demands' in the context of the 'demands and capacities model' in Chapter 2.

When we consider these behaviours, it is all too easy to do so from a judgemental position. We believe that instead we should be trying to understand the meaning of the behaviours for the parents. If they jump in with answers, might it be construed from their point of view as a caring and protective way of showing their concern that their child is not hurt? If they look away, is it so the child does not see they are upset? If they tell the child to stop, is it from a belief that the stammering is deliberate and can be controlled? In order to help a parent to change these behaviours we need to be accepting, to suspend our own judgement, and empathise with the parent (Rogers, 1957). We also need to have a subsuming construct system. Kelly (1991, p28) described this as: 'a system which is primarily methodological and which will therefore permit the therapist to deal with individuals who themselves vary widely in their personal-construct systems'.

Family interaction

Observing the pattern of communication within the family gives us a context for the dysfluency. Some of the following may be useful questions for the clinician to try to answer as she increases her understanding of how family dynamics are played out in verbal interactions:

◆ Who is good/bad at listening?
◆ Who initiates/controls conversations?
◆ Who is listened to/not listened to?
◆ Are there rules about turn taking or is there a verbal 'free for all'?
◆ Are there communication patterns in the family – who talks to whom and what about?
◆ Are there quiet and noisy family members; how is our client construed?
◆ Are there silent times in conversations?
◆ How much interrupting goes on?
◆ Which people in the family does the child get on with/not get on with/enjoy/not enjoy spending time with?
◆ When are the family together? What do they enjoy doing? Do they like talking? Is the television usually on?
◆ Do the family eat together? Is this enjoyable, or is there friction over what/how they eat?

Discipline

In understanding parents and children, it can be useful to look at the way discipline is seen and carried out. Turner & Helms (1991) suggested that there are three main styles of parental discipline which are, in fact, often mixed. *Authoritarian* parents see obedience and control as important in their attempts to enforce desired behaviour. *Authoritative* parents are also concerned with directing behaviour, but give explanations and are more prepared to negotiate. *Permissive* parents, on the other hand, do not aim to control and rarely use sanctions, but prefer to consult. Attitudes to discipline may vary both within and between parents. Understanding the family's view on discipline and the way in which they deal with problems gives the clinician more insight into understanding both how the family function and how they might deal with the 'problem of dysfluency'. We are not aiming to create 'ideal' families, but rather to help families cope more effectively in a way that can make sense to them and can be growth-enhancing, rather than growth-restricting, for its members.

Busyness of household/time spent together

Some families conduct their lives in a leisurely manner; some others seem to be in a continual rush in which there is an underlying 'hurry-up' message. While many households have periods when everyone has a lot to do in a limited time (for example, getting ready for school and work in the morning), for some the pressure seems to be almost continual. Dysfluent children in such a household often seem to feel a need to do things, including speaking, at speed. Linked in with this is the question of how much time the parents spend with their children and what happens in this time. Rustin (1987) asks parents of younger children to spend 3–5 minutes per day on four to seven occasions a week in a 'verbally participative event' of the child's choosing. This is used as an observation and learning task for the parents. In our clinical experience, we have noted how difficult it is for many parents to find even this very limited amount of time to spend without a specific agenda.

Cultural issues

In our work with dysfluent children, we inevitably come across people from a variety of cultures. If we are to understand the dysfluency in the context of children and their families, we must therefore aim to understand any cultural implications that the dysfluency may hold. In helping the child and/or the family to reconstrue the dysfluency, we should be trying not to negate the cultural perspectives, but rather to work within them. We should not impose our construing of dysfluency on the family, but instead aim to help them to discover if there are any other ways of coping that do not conflict with their beliefs. If we are told that eating 'tanda' or cold food makes the child more dysfluent and hence the child is not allowed ice cream (as may be the case in some Asian cultures), we accept that this is one of the ways in which they see the problem and are trying to help (and who is to say that it is not as acceptable a viewpoint as any other?). We may encourage them to test out their hypothesis (eg introduce more hot foods or 'garam' as a balance) and look at whether there may be other possibilities and solutions that they may find equally helpful.

Religious events or ceremonies that include a 'performance' element may also put extra demands on a dysfluent young person. A confirmation or first communion service may require a child to make certain responses at exactly the right moment. The Jewish bar mitzvah demands both a reading in Hebrew and a speech in English. Young people can understandably find the build-up to such occasions a considerable ordeal. To stammer in front of one's friends and family in such a public gathering may feel like one's worst nightmare come true.

Change and other issues

Many children have to deal with several changes in their lives. Some children have to cope with an enormous amount of change in a short space of time. Although many appear to take this in their stride, others do not have the capacity to deal with the demands that even relatively minor changes may place on them. Most children will have to learn to be away from their mothers, with a childminder, at nursery or at school. Many will have to deal with the birth of a new baby and all the attendant associated anxiety. Others have to be admitted to hospital or move house in their early years. Nowadays children also experience such events as a parent being made redundant, or parents quarrelling or separating. Some may be faced with the death of a close relative, especially a grandparent. While there appears to be little empirical research in this area, Peters & Guitar (1991) have pointed out that increased dysfluency often appears to accompany the stress and tension of particular life events in all children. A study by Rustin & Purser (1991) of 209 dysfluent children between the ages of 5 and 13 years found significant health and emotional problems in many of the parents and children. Yairi & Ambrose (1992b) looked at the onset of dysfluency in 87 pre-school children and reported that 43 per cent of their parents reported emotional or physical stress factors at some point before the onset. As no control group of non-stuttering children was examined for such factors, it is not possible to comment on how significant these factors might be. An additional point to consider is that although parents may often report the onset of dysfluency as occurring at such times, one might ask if sometimes this is linked to a natural search for an identifiable cause. Some of our adult clients have indeed told us categorically that they started to stammer at the time of a particular trauma. When this has been checked out with family members, we sometimes discover that the dysfluency had been present in a mild form before the event.

A further area for consideration is child abuse. In our counselling of adults, we have seen a number of clients who have disclosed to us incidents of previous abuse, both physical and sexual. Often, the adult will construe the stammer as being closely connected with the abuse; the dysfluency may indeed have started at around the same time as the abuse. Issues of control, of secrecy and of hiding can have particular relevance in such cases. When we are working with children we must be aware of any clues that suggest the possibility that there has been abuse.

THE IMPORTANCE OF THE INDIVIDUAL

Having considered the context of the dysfluency, we now turn our attention to the individual child. While we have some views about the nature of stammering and factors that affect its development, it is important not to let those presumptions colour our view of the individual. Children present in different ways, with problems and issues that are special to them. We must be open to the possibilities that fall outside the generalities found in the literature. We must be credulous listeners and believe what children and parents report, seeing the difficulties from their point of view, rather than from the perspective of the textbook. What do we want to know about children? How will the things we find out help us decide whether their dysfluency is more or less likely to be, or to develop into, a more serious problem?

Issues to Consider in the Individual Child

Children's attitude to their speech

We are interested in understanding to what children attribute their dysfluency. Do they see it as something that 'happens' to them, over which they have no control? Or is it seen as something that they 'do' and consequently a behaviour it is possible to change or control? It is noteworthy that change to a more internal locus of control was found to be one of the significant factors in the prediction of long-term outcome in a study of adults by Andrews & Craig (1988).

Fluency disrupters

Fluency disrupters can be thought of as behavioural manifestations of some of the environmental 'demands' that we will refer to in our discussion of the demands and capacities model in Chapter 2. The clinician's awareness of these will be helpful when working with parents as they change some of the factors that affect their child's ability to balance demands and capacities. It is, however, necessary to be aware that the behaviours themselves are not the only important factors. Hayhow & Levy (1989, p59) warn us to consider 'the importance of understanding personal meanings and not just cataloguing behaviours or observed events'.

Fluency disrupters can be divided into two categories: factors within children and factors in the environment. Those within children may be physical (such as tiredness, illness), linguistic (such as complexity of utterance), emotional (such as excitement, upset, urgency of the communication) or cognitive (such as the need to express oneself verbally and to sustain interest). External factors involve the way others react to the dysfluency (such as saying 'slow down', looking away), reactions to verbal communication (such as interrupting, excessive questioning, correction of errors of pronunciation or grammar, complexity of adults' speech), or general factors in the home (such as competition for talking time, sibling rivalry, poor listening, time pressure, noise levels, high or low expectations, discipline). We will look at these factors in more detail later in the book, particularly their relevance to specific categories: early, borderline and confirmed dysfluency.

Impact of stammering

If we take the personal construct psychology view, we must accept that children behave in a particular way because that behaviour has meaning for them. Our aim must therefore be to understand the individual meaning for each child. We need to consider which aspects of a child's behaviour help us to understand whether and how much the dysfluency is troubling him. Signs of avoidance, for example, show us that a child is construing his dysfluency as unacceptable and therefore as something not to be shown. Avoidance comes in all shapes and forms: circumlocution, difficulty in finding words, saying as little as possible, giving up on/shortening an utterance, saying 'I don't know', using starters or fillers and word substitution. These behaviours are less common in younger children, but they are by no means rare. One child, aged three, whom we knew would refer to himself as 'this boy', rather than use his name. Another, aged two and a half, would actually change the subject when he became stuck on a particular word.

Children's use of eye contact can be another clue as to their feelings about the dysfluency. If they look away during a dysfluent utterance, we may presume some concern on their behalf. Starkweather (1987) made an interesting observation regarding such behaviour, suggesting that it often occurs in response to a similar behaviour in the parent. If the parent breaks eye contact with the child when he is dysfluent, the child may learn to do the same.

Perkins (1992) suggested that dysfluency can have 'pay-offs' (albeit at an unconscious level) for children, which in fact increase the likelihood of its development. Some of these may be positive, such as more time and attention, less discipline, or being allowed to interrupt. Others may be negative, such as being told to stop or slow down, or an adult's reaction of distress and concern. Perkins argues that both sorts can be 'addictive', as they can become powerful ways for children to gain attention and control. Some of Perkins' assertions about the nature of stammering are contentious and not backed up by any research findings (for example, he suggests that it is primarily caused by 'a dominance conflict about being assertive'). However, there is certainly food for thought for clinicians in considering what purpose the dysfluency may serve for children and their families.

Hayhow & Levy (1989) point out the need for the clinician to explore the child's construing of the dysfluency in order to discover whether he is using a 'stuttering-fluency' construct to make sense of his world. They offer a variety of exploratory techniques to use with children of all ages. We will discuss these and other ideas in Chapter 7.

THE THERAPIST'S APPROACH

Understanding Dysfluency

When we consider dysfluency, we start from a position of not knowing. We do not know its cause, although we might speculate from the many available theories. We think we know a little about its nature, although the evidence is conflicting and what we think we know today may be disproved tomorrow. We even believe at times that we have some of the answers; that our current understanding of stammering is *the* understanding, our current way of working *the* way of working. We have only to look back over the past few decades to realise how foolish this kind of thinking can be. If we accept that we actually know very little and therefore we cannot be experts, we are more open to new ideas and new evidence, and can more easily reject ideas that no longer make sense to us. We can be scientists in the Kellian sense, forming and reforming hypotheses, making predictions and reacting according to the results of our experiments.

Client-Centred Philosophy

While we have acknowledged the need to take several factors into consideration when painting a picture of children's communication contexts, this does not detract from our client-centred philosophy. Our primary focus is always on individual children, although we will be aware of what is around them. We will believe a child's view of the world and, indeed, aim to see this view ourselves 'as if' standing in their shoes. This means, in practical terms, using credulous listening and being open to alternative perspectives. At times children's views can be different from those around them and, given the variability that stammering can have, this is not an uncommon situation. For example, the child may see his stammer as severe and impacting greatly on his life, while his parents comment, 'it is hardly there at all' and of 'no real significance'. Conversely, it may be the parents who perceive a problem whereas the child perceives a minor inconvenience. In such situations, it is important not to set these different views in opposition, but to act as a facilitator for each of the parties to see the other's perspective.

Choice

One of the aspects of speech and language therapy that differentiates it from the interventions of some independent practitioners is the issue of 'tailor made' as opposed to 'off the peg' intervention. As qualified speech & language therapists, we are able to assess each client fully and make a professional decision on the types of intervention best suited to their individual needs. The other aspect of our management is the negotiation that takes place between the client/carer and the therapist regarding the processes, so once again the individuality of the intervention is ensured. This 'tailoring' to suit the individual and the discussion of therapy, functions to empower the client and give them a sense of choice and responsibility. We believe this is especially important with respect to dysfluency, a disorder that can impose feelings of lack of choice and control. While this negotiation can be harder to undertake with young children, it is nevertheless an important principle.

Non-Expert Stance

Finally, we are aware that many families come to us seeking the advice and opinion of the 'expert'. While we do have some information of use to them, it is important not to set ourselves apart from them and the issues of concern. We believe that *they* are actually the expert in their particular situation and know their child much better than we will ever do. Thus we need to enlist their help, and to act as partners in a collaborative problem-solving approach with the child and the family. We discuss the factors that seem to be worrying them and together try and identify possible solutions. In this way the family are not deskilled, but learn a process of resolving difficulties that may be of use to them in the future.

Our approach is integrative. We draw on a wide variety of techniques and approaches, but we believe that whatever we do must be underpinned by theory and research, and not just a haphazard conglomeration of ideas and intuitions.

CONCLUSION

In this chapter, we have set the scene for much of what will follow in this book. We have considered dysfluency in general terms, and how it might be presented to us at the start of our management in the form of a referral. We have gone on to look at some basic principles of the management of dysfluent children and have explored in more detail several issues to be included in a case-history format. These are summarised in Handout 2 at the end of the chapter. In other chapters, we will discuss factors specific to each stage of stammering. As we look at these, we must always remind ourselves that we are concerned with individual children in individual environments. We do not want to end up as fact gatherers who diagnose in terms of the numbers of items we can tick off on our checklists. Rather, we need to be asking what the information is telling us about its personal meaningfulness for those we are seeing. Information itself is of no use; it is how it helps us to make sense of the child and his dysfluency that is important.

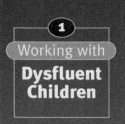

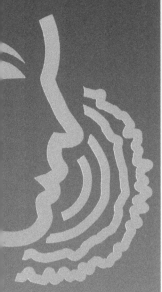

HANDOUT: PRIORITISATION CHECKLIST

Name

Date

Issues	Present	Absent
Expression of anxiety by child, parent/carer or other professional		
Identification of 'a problem' by child, parent, professional (including the label of 'stammer')		
Avoidance behaviours, and development of other covert features in the child		
Teasing or bullying of child by peer group		
Modifications or changes to child's speech		
Presence of struggle or increased tension in child during or in anticipation of speech		
Feeling by child of being out of control during speaking		
Communication/situational anxiety which may be anticipated by the child or present in the child during the event		
Inability of child to say what he wants to say when he wants to say it		
Specific behaviour and/or communication changes in child		
Family history of stammering		

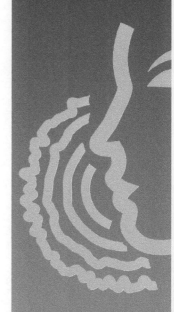
HANDOUT: IDEAS FOR INCLUSION IN CASE HISTORY FOR CHILDREN WHO ARE DYSFLUENT

Name _____

Date _____

HOLISTIC MANAGEMENT		NOTES
Significant others	Emotions	
	Attitude to speech	
	Attitude to dysfluency	
	Function of dysfluency	
	Listening	
Family dynamics	Interactions	
	Listening	
	Discipline	
	Busyness of household	
	Change	
	Other problems	
Cultural issues		

THE INDIVIDUAL CHILD		NOTES
Fluency disrupters	Attitude to speech	
	Internal factors	
	External factors	
Impact of dysfluency	Awareness	
	'Pay offs'	

CLINICIAN'S APPROACH	NOTES
How do you understand this child's dysfluency?	
How is your approach client-centred?	
How can you create choice in this child's life?	
How were you able to give a non-expert opinion?	

BASIC PRINCIPLES

Development of Stammering

In terms of current thinking we owe much to a number of early theorists such as Johnson, Bloodstein and Van Riper. There are echoes of their work running through models in common use today. Of particular significance is the congruence that all the experts exhibit in identifying a number of key factors in the development of stammering:

◆ The nature and frequency of children's non-fluencies

◆ Children's own attitudes to their fluent and non-fluent speech

◆ The reaction of significant other people to children's speech

◆ Children's emotional reaction to attitudes to their speech and attitudes of significant other people in the environment

◆ Children's development, including speech and language skills

◆ Environmental pressures.

While theories apportion weight to these factors differently, there is general agreement as to their importance. Currently, following the work of Yairi and others, the nature of children's speech patterns is the subject of attention. This, and other significant factors, will be considered in detail in the next chapter.

When we start looking for hard evidence or concrete facts in terms of knowledge and understanding of the development of stammering, we are disappointed. Although there is a plethora of research in the area, much of it is contradictory and/or inconclusive. As clinicians, we would seem to have to start from a position of 'not knowing', which can be a problem for those wishing to operate from an expert stance.

So where does this leave clinicians who are required to work from an evidence base? We urge clinicians not to discard contradictory research, but rather to analyse and assimilate opinions from a wide range of evidence. This will include evidence of all types (qualitative, quantitative, reviews of specific areas, single case studies, and so on), textbook information, views of experienced clinicians, client and carer opinion and clinicians' own experience. We also would encourage clinicians to draw on their knowledge and experience from associated areas to assist them in their clinical decision making. For example, there is much evidence in the field of parent-child interaction that can be usefully gleaned from areas such as semantic-pragmatic disorders, social skills programmes, learning disabilities – and, indeed, adults who stammer.

The Balancing Act

We now turn our attention to theoretical models that reflect the research to date. The literature on stammering currently includes a model that appears to synthesise what we know about dysfluency in children. Since our description in the first edition of *Working with Dysfluent Children*, we have come to think of and describe it as 'the scales model' but for those who are unfamiliar with our image we repeat it here. Imagine a set of old-fashioned kitchen scales, the type that uses brass weights to counter-balance the weight of the substance being weighed. The child's speech is represented by the scales: tip the balance one way and he is fluent; overload in the opposite direction and his speech becomes non-fluent.

This idea of imbalance was a concern of Joseph Sheehan (1970, 1975) and was also discussed in 1964 by Andrews & Harris in their survey conducted in Newcastle. Twenty years later, the idea was followed up by Starkweather (1981, 1985) and in 1987, in his book *Fluency and Stuttering*, he formally described what he called the 'demands and capacities' model (Figure 1).

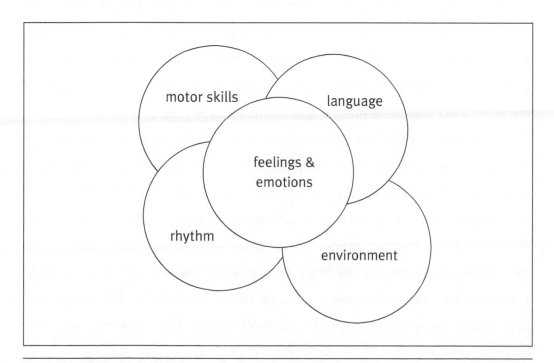

Figure 1
Components of the demands and capacities model

Model or theory?

Interestingly, Starkweather does not regard the demands and capacities model as a theory in the pure sense, but more a way of attempting to make some sense of what are, as we have seen, often contradictory pieces of evidence. The demands and capacities model looks at what we know about speech and language production and the development of speech and language in young children, and tries to explain and then integrate the existing information.

The model has two fundamental premises:

1   'The child's growing capacity to talk more easily is paralleled by increasing demands for fluent speech, demands placed on the children by the people they communicate with and by themselves.'

2   'When the child's capacity for fluency exceeds the demands, the child will talk fluently, but when the child lacks the capacity to meet demands for fluency, stuttering or something like it will occur.' (1987, p75)

Thus Starkweather states that we know children become increasingly fluent with age; we can observe the slow laboured searching for words in toddlers and contrast this with the comparative flow of language that is produced only a few years later. In a relatively short space of time, most children develop the ability to cope with expressing themselves in quite long sentences, using a wealth of vocabulary and in a manner that is appropriate to the situation. They also seem to develop a number of strategies to cope with any hesitancies, pauses or other lapses in fluency. Starkweather argues that this growing ability to talk is based upon several capacities and that these are the fundamental building blocks for fluent speech. Paralleling this development, Starkweather believes, are a set of demands that can be self-imposed by children, or generated by their environment and those around them. These demands change and often increase as children get older; for example, most adults will use a slower rate of speaking with young children, whereas older children are required to decode speech at an increasingly faster rate as they themselves age. Generally, the majority of children are able to cope with these pressures. Their capacities progress and develop in line with the demands placed upon them. However, there are some children for whom this is not the case; either their capacities are not able to keep pace or the demands placed upon the system are too great. The resulting imbalance is the cause of the breakdown in fluent speech production. Starkweather goes on to say that, when these resulting breakdowns in fluency occur, children may respond with struggle and increased tension, which becomes the automatic pattern associated with stammering.

Table 1 summarises the many aspects of interactive behaviours that can influence a child's dysfluency.

DEMANDS AND CAPACITIES

The list of demands and capacities cited by Starkweather is a useful one, and corresponds well to most clinicians' views of important factors. We recommend readers to his text (Starkweather, 1987) for a fuller discussion of the clinical research data that substantiates his points. We will briefly outline his list and, in this edition of *Working with Dysfluent Children*, will detail our own thinking in this area over recent times, indicating the advantages and pitfalls we have experienced in our use of this model.

Capacities

Ability to control movements in the vocal tract

Under this point, four main areas are considered important:

1 Children must be able to react to a stimulus; to recognise the stimulus as one which requires a response, and then to react to it rapidly and appropriately.

2 Children need the ability to coordinate movements of different parts of the vocal tract that are occurring simultaneously. For example, when producing the *b* in 'boy', a child must be able to initiate and sustain the movements of the laryngeal muscles required for phonation, at the same time making a bilabial lip seal for the closure phase of the plosive, and release the closure at the correct moment, given sufficient air pressure for the release phase of the sound.

3 It is necessary for movements to be planned and executed in a sequence appropriate for the production of a word or series of words.

Table 1 Checklist of interactive behaviour

Scale		
1 ◄─────────────── 5 ──────────────► 10		
Eye contact		Poor and/or inappropriate eye contact
Turn taking, appropriate speaking window		Interrupting, rushing child's turn, completing his sentences/words

Positive feedback:
    Verbal – praise & reinforcement
    Non-verbal – positive facial expression, body posture, and so on
		Negative feedback:
		    Verbal – negative criticism
		    Non-verbal – negative facial expression, tense body posture, and so on

Friendly vocal tone Acceptance of dysfluency		Unfriendly, non-encouraging tone of voice Suggestions of speech modifications
Openness about stammering		No discussion of dysfluent speech
Moderated rate of parental speech		Fast rate of parental speech
Use of pausing		Lack of pausing
Appropriate language level used (vocabulary, sentence length, complexity of ideas expressed)		Inappropriate language level used (too low or too high)
Open-ended questions		Too many and too direct questions
Lack of demand/performance speech		Child required to perform in speaking terms
Balance of time spent talking and listening		Parent talks too much, monopolises the conversation. Child does too much listening
Parent following child's lead in topic and change		Parental choice of topic and timing of change of topic
Quality talking time		Little or no time for talking together
Use of humour		Little or no humour in interaction
Appropriate physical contact		Little or no physical contact
Appropriate space		Crowding or too much distance from child
Parent follows up on previous information/topic initiated by child		Little or no follow-up on information/topic initiated by child
Child encouraged to contribute his opinions		Child not encouraged and/or contributions to conversation not valued
Parent controls distractions in the environment, such as television		Distractions allowed to block communication

4 A child must also have a system whereby he monitors all of the above and puts in place a repair process if and when his abilities break down and/or errors occur. For example, if the sequence of phonemes within a sentence or phrase is incorrect, then the child must recognise the error and correct it in order to convey the appropriate meaning: 'Can I have a boclate chiscuit, please?' (chocolate biscuit).

Rhythm

This is an area about which little is known, but it is Starkweather's belief that possession of a sense of rhythm contributes to children's capacities for fluent speech. He argues that rhythm enables children to anticipate movements in speech production and that this ability to predict what should occur, or is about to occur, will contribute to children's feelings of control and confidence in a speaking situation. We know from studies of early language development that children develop this sense from experimentation at a pre-verbal stage. They are reported to play with different intonation patterns, often for long periods at a time. It would be interesting to follow those children who did not carry out these 'experiments' with tone and sound to see if their subsequent rhythmical skills, including their capacity to anticipate movements of speech, were in any way impaired. We wonder if these early silent children already have the scales tipped in favour of non-fluent speech.

Clinically we are aware that some, but not all, children who have dysfluent speech present with poor rhythmical skills. As with other aspects of the demands and capacities model, we are not concerned with causation, and certainly would not suggest that poor rhythmical skills cause stammering. However, as with other aspects in the scales, help in this area may be one factor that assists children to improve their capacity to be more fluent.

In considering what abilities children should possess to develop an appropriate sense of rhythm, we have identified a number of prerequisites:

◆ Hear the sound (that is, listen and attend to it)
◆ Discriminate (that is, separate it from other sounds in the environment [sound/ground] and understand its tones, pitch and so on as different from other sounds).

Then, moving on to consider abilities required to identify rhythm, children need to attend to the sound(s) in specific ways:

◆ Duration of the sound
◆ The number of repetitions of the sound
◆ The sequence of the sound and no sound (that is, silence intervals)
◆ The spacing of sound and silence.

Feelings & emotions

Although in the first edition of *Working with Dysfluent Children* this section related to children's emotional development, we are now extending it to include the way in which children's emotional being or predisposition interacts with their environment, including people and situations. We know that more emotionally mature children are able to cope in strange, unfamiliar and threatening situations. Children who are less emotionally and socially developed may become anxious and hesitant in these circumstances. In terms of capacities for fluent speech, Starkweather & Gottwald (1990) regard the following as important areas for assessment:

◆ Levels of independence
◆ Subordination of immediate needs
◆ Crying
◆ Ability to share with peers and siblings.

Other researchers and clinicians have included other aspects of the child within this category. Riley & Riley (1983) discussed the high self-expectations for performance that children who stutter appear to have. In addition, Oyler & Ramig (1995) found these children to be more 'sensitive'. This sensitivity was defined as emotional susceptibility and reactivity, and susceptibility to noise, stress, time, pressure, and physical pain.

A table of possible disrupting factors was listed by Hill (1999) and includes two main issues. The first concerns low tolerance, including gaining listener attention, urgency about communication, attempting difficult tasks, and the child not having his own way. The second main concern is behavioural characteristics, and this includes difficulty making transitions, being uncomfortable in new situations, risk taking and impulsivity, attention seeking, and being perceptive/observant.

The issue of self-esteem

Much is written about the connection between stammering and self-esteem. In the literature there seems to be a 'double-edged' hypothesis: a child has low self-esteem because he stammers (Bardrick & Sheehan, 1956) or a child stammers because he has low self-esteem. Sheehan & Martyn (1966) stated that individuals who view themselves as 'stammerers' are less likely to recover spontaneously. In contrast, in a recent study Yovetich *et al* (2000) found no difference on a five-dimensional measure of self-esteem between school-age children who stutter and their fluent counterparts. Woods (1974) also found that, although a school child may rate himself as a poor speaker, his view of himself in terms of social standing with classmates may remain unaffected.

This research illustrates the complexity of this issue. It is our view that it is not a simple matter of identifying certain characteristics, such as self-esteem, and then labelling a child who displays these features as a child who is at risk of stammering. We cannot say that excitable children are at risk of stammering; the fact that we know, and indeed have in our respective families, excitable children who have not developed dysfluent speech, proves the point. Similarly, not all children who are lacking in confidence or self-esteem will stammer.

The importance of construing fluency

Our hypothesis is that children with persistent stammering have in some way allowed their stammering behaviour and their own and/or other people's reactions to their stammering to affect aspects of them as individuals.

Arguably, the years of childhood are about the mastery of skills, the establishment of varying degrees of control over our bodily functions, general motor and social behaviour, emotions, and so on. In that process we all experience difficulties with a particular skill, behaviour or some aspect of learning. Indeed, one of us (TS) was a late swimmer, and did not experience real pleasure in the act of swimming until my late 20s. The point here is that this is a natural process – however, how we construe these difficulties and how we see ourselves as a consequence is much more important. In some situations the fact that I was a non-swimming teenager was socially isolating and contributed to my construction of myself as 'not sporty'. However, it did not affect my belief that I was intelligent, creative, and a bit thin! I did not make choices about my social interactions or my circle of friends because I was unable to swim at that time. Later I had different experiences, such as learning to play squash and badminton, which helped me reconstrue myself as someone who enjoyed sporting activities.

Children experiencing speech difficulties may react the same way – that is, their stammering speech does not have an impact on who they believe themselves to be and/or what they think they can and cannot achieve. However, there are some children who present differently. It is not the difference itself which is isolating, but a child's reaction to it. For such children their experience of 'bumpy talking' is highly significant and 'stigmatising', and it devalues them in other aspects of their life. They are acutely aware of their different speech and this awareness may isolate them socially. Learning new skills and developing in other ways may not be perceived as an enriching experience for these children, but rather may serve to highlight the inadequacies in their communication ('I may be good at maths but if only I was good at talking I could answer the questions in class').

In contrast, children who construe dysfluent speech as something separate that does not have an impact on other aspects of their lives are less likely to develop covert issues such as guilt, shame, anger and anxiety. Their different talking is like the differences they encounter in others (she's good at football/not good at football; he likes pasta/doesn't like pasta) and does not mean anything fundamental about them as individuals. Other behaviours, learning and their development in other areas are not seen in relation to their talking ('I am good at maths, not as good at reading out loud in English, but I'm still going to try for a part in the school play because drama is fun!').

In the context of the demands and capacities model, we look at aspects of children's construing of their talking that could be regarded as positive. For example:

- Having a perspective on speaking which does not spill over into other behaviours.
- Accepting strengths and weaknesses.
- Devaluing skills that are not as strong as other skills, for example, 'I'm hopeless at art, but it doesn't matter because I just want to do it as a hobby'.
- Making decisions that take account of the whole person, for example, 'I'm going to Rachel's party, because she looks good and we might play kiss catch!' as opposed to, 'I'm not going to Rachel's party, because my speech will be bumpy if I try and talk to her and everyone will laugh when they hear me'.
- Not being a perfectionist. Being able to tolerate mistakes and accepting errors as part of a learning process.
- Believing that the content and/or the message are more important than the delivery.
- Openness about speech.

Starkweather is very specific about what he means concerning this last point. He believes that children's ability to talk about non-fluencies is an important capacity. He argues that if children have good metalinguistic skills and are able to describe the process of talking in a way which helps them understand and make some sense of it, then this capacity will work in their favour.

We have some sympathy with this standpoint, and have experience of it working in our family and professional lives. Alastair, a child of one of the authors (TS), experienced a particularly difficult non-fluent period at about two and a half years of age. He would repeat long strings of syllables and words for some considerable time. His awareness of his difficulty was demonstrated one mealtime when he asked for a drink: 'Mummy I want ju ju ju ju ju ju ju – Oh! [frustrated] I can't say that. You say it Mummy!' He knew exactly what he wanted to say, had identified the lexical item correctly, but could not produce the word in its entirety. He had also monitored his own production and knew that the production was incomplete and therefore unacceptable to him. However, he was able to convey his frustration to his parent and ask for help. (In terms of managing non-fluency in children generally, this situation was a valuable experience for Mum! She was able to discuss with the child how sometimes words get stuck and it was nothing to be worried about. It seemed appropriate to make such a comment in this situation, but the response of the carer should always take into account the awareness of the child.) Compare this example with the case of *C*, a child who came to see us with severe blocks or prolongations at two years of age. His non-fluencies were of a different type, but still disrupted his communication in the same way as Alastair's, lasting several seconds. *C* appeared aware of his problem too, but managed it by changing his sentences entirely, including changing the subject and stopping talking altogether. At one point his parents came to the clinic after a difficult weekend when *C* had behaved uncharacteristically. He had appeared unhappy and withdrawn, communicating very little and preferring solitary occupations. It was our view that *C* was aware of the problems with his speech, but did not have the strategies to deal with them. Had his metalinguistic capacities been more advanced, then Starkweather would argue that *C* may have been one step closer coming to terms with his non-fluencies.

We believe that children's construing of their non-fluent speech has an important part to play in the development of stammering, and will discuss this in some detail in Chapter 3.

Demands

According to the model, demands placed upon a child's fluency potential come from two main areas:

1 Demands placed on the child's language skills
2 Demands that originate from the child's environment.

We would also suggest a third area:

3 Demands that a child may place upon himself which are therefore internal in origin.

We will look at each of these areas in turn.

Development of language skills

Each aspect of language can impose its own pressures on children's fluency, as we will see.

Syntax   As syntactical skills develop, sentences increase in length and complexity. Children are then required to plan and execute longer sequences that have a more complex organisation and structure. In any communication process the response, planning and execution time is limited. Children have to create these mature constructions or utterances with no extra time. Thus they perceive they have to produce these more difficult sentences in the same time taken to produce the less complex ones. While increasing the length of utterance, a child must simultaneously develop an ability to move parts of the vocal tract with increasing speed and agility.

Semantics   Next there are the pressures arising from semantic development. As the child's language skills progress, he has a greater number of lexical items and different semantic fields from which to make a selection. This makes word choice more difficult and potentially more time consuming. However, to accompany this process, most children develop an increasing capacity to match a lexical item to the meaning they wish to convey. This word-finding and word-matching ability must mature alongside semantic development if speech is to possess the characteristics of fluent speech.

Phonology   Once again, the increased length and sequences of words are demanding of children's motor skills. In addition, we know that some of the phonological processes in more mature form require an increase in length; for example, younger children will reduce the consonant-consonant-consonant-vowel form at the beginning of a string to consonant-vowel or consonant-consonant-vowel. With maturity, they are able to give the cluster of consonants its full value and cope with the planning and execution of the sequence. Consequently, developing phonological processes creates demands upon children's planning of sequences of speech and, possibly more importantly for fluency, makes demands on speed of motor speech patterns.

Pragmatics   The demands of developing pragmatic skills are summarised by Starkweather as two factors:

1   Diminishing spontaneity
2   Increasing need to control the form and content of language.

There is much documentary evidence supporting the concept of spontaneity. As parents, we have seen the process in our own children: the gradual move from externalising all their thoughts in a play situation, for example, to selecting only those aspects they wish to make comment on or those they think their listeners or playmates would be interested in hearing. We recall how our own children talked when playing with a train set. At first we heard the whole sequence of play, beginning with the train setting off, then going through the tunnel, up the hill and finally arriving at the station to pick up and deposit passengers. In later years, the children drew our attention only to those aspects of play considered important enough: 'Look, Mummy, the train's crashed!' With the appearance of appropriate turn-taking behaviour, this spontaneity is further inhibited as the child has to retain the utterance until it is his turn to speak.

Older children also have to cope with the demands of certain situations or individuals, as will be discussed shortly. However, there are demands made on their pragmatic skills that may be specific to these situations or people. An example is of Thomas, who loves computer games. When asked about the latest game by a chum or friendly adult, he is quite vociferous in his description and may include much detail. Should the same question be asked by an elderly aunt who he perceives to be a non-user of computers, then he would alter his reply to account for her lack of knowledge and, perhaps, lack of real interest. So, with age, children can alter the content of their language in line with their views or perceptions about listeners. They also initiate communication, use questions more and are able to take the lead in conversations. This demonstrates that children are able to take more responsibility for communication as their language skills progress.

The environment

Children do not exist in a vacuum. There are demands that originate from the people with whom they communicate and situations in which they find themselves. We consider the family, peer groups and school to be the key areas. In line with what we discussed in the section on communication dynamics in Chapter 1, we believe that there is a connection between the speech children hear and the speech they themselves produce. There is evidence to suggest that children try to emulate the speech of those around them; if that is the case, then the language levels used, the rate of speech, and turn-taking behaviour are very important. Again we make the point we made previously, that these aspects of speech production should be seen, not in isolation, but as parts of the interaction.

Language levels of significant others   The levels of language used by adults may be syntactically too complicated, the vocabulary beyond children's understanding, and the sentences too long to be retained. Similarly, children may play with a peer group who use language beyond their capacities. Children may be struggling to comprehend communication and in terms of expressive speech, struggling to copy structures and vocabulary that are too sophisticated for their developmental ability.

Speech rate of significant others   As we have already noted, adults tend to increase their rate of speech as children grow older. When others use a faster speech rate, more is demanded of children in terms of speed of decoding, retention and time given to formulate, process and produce their own responses. We must consider whether demands of speed are beyond children's neuromuscular, cognitive and social or emotional response capacities. We must also think whether or not particular children are likely to be affected by a faster rate of speech than they themselves can produce. Will they notice and be aware of the difference? Will they try and compensate for it and increase their own rate accordingly? If they increase their rate and become dysfluent as a result, how will the adult in the dyad respond: by slowing down, looking away, telling them to 'slow down'?

Dynamics of turn-taking behaviours   The issue of rate of speech is linked with turn-taking behaviours. Very often, adults and older siblings who use faster rates of speech exhibit rapid turn-taking. Conversation in such families is quick-fire comment and response, and children can feel that there is little time to say what they wish to say, and may feel they have reduced time to break into and initiate their contribution. Sometimes conversation in families can be dominated by older, more accomplished, articulate individuals, with children perceiving they have no valued part to play. Given such a scenario, it is important to consider how children react to the situation. Some children withdraw and learn not to risk their fluency in this competitive environment; others become angry and may lash out at the older sibling in frustration.

Feelings of urgency   There may be a general sense of 'hurriedness'. The family or classroom activities may be carried out in a rushed, perhaps frenzied way, with the children urged to hurry up and get on to the next activity. In such circumstances, children may have feelings of urgency and generalise these to talking. Thus they may feel that there is little time for planning speech and that they have to speak at an accelerated pace, to produce what they have to say before everyone moves on and their point is lost.

Social demands

There are also social demands that exert pressure on children's ability to be fluent. This type of demand can be linked to a particular person, such as the relative who bombards children with questions, or may be linked to a specific situation, such as a large family gathering. Again, we would be keen to know how children who attend our clinics respond to these pressures and what coping strategies, if any, they have.

Demand speech   As parents we have been aware of demanding speech from our children perhaps at inappropriate times, often fulfilling our own need to know rather than the children's desire to communicate. An example of this would be meeting children from school; we are keen to learn about how they have spent the day, what topics have been covered in class, who they played with and whether or not they ate their lunch! We do not *need* to know all this information, or in fact any of it, immediately, but we ask anyway. Looking at the situation from the children's perspective, they have just completed a full and tiring day when demands of various types were placed upon them, and now a whole new set is presented by parents. This demand for speech at certain times or by certain people, transforms children into performers rather than spontaneous speakers, and the demands may outweigh children's abilities or wishes to talk.

Family dynamics   Starkweather & Gottwald (1990) also discuss another type of demand in which families demand too much of children socially. They quote examples of children acting as interpreters for parents or adopting a 'go-between' role during marital discord. Both roles carry enormous responsibilities and may prove too much of a burden for many children. Any assessment of social demand should be made comparatively with children's social maturity, including confidence and degree of social skill.

Emotional demands

Demands upon children's emotions come from a variety of sources.

Events   Certain activities or events act positively to heighten emotion, such as birthday parties, religious festivals, or visiting relatives and friends.

Sources of negative emotion   There are those less positive situations that upset, alarm and perhaps threaten children's emotional stability. Stress events for adults have been well documented and include moving house, changing jobs, being made redundant, marriage, divorce, death, birth, and so on. For children, a similar list may include moving house, changing schools, losing friends or a precious toy, the arrival of a new baby, death of a parent, relative or close friend, illness, marital discord and divorce. All or any of these events can result in increased tension.

Reactions to non-fluency from others   Non-fluency itself is also a very emotive area. It may produce reactions in others that children find difficult to understand and manage.

◆ Parents or carers may increase the amount of attention they give during moments of non-fluency (for example, immediately turn and face children or attend to them for longer periods). Thus children perceive that the quantity and quality of attention they receive is greater when they are non-fluent.

◆ Listeners will respond with subtle, non-verbal messages that convey to children that their speech is unacceptable (for example, lose eye contact, alter their posture or seating position, freeze, turn away or change the subject, all of which tell children: 'Your talking is bad. I don't like it').

◆ Some people are more direct (for example, they instruct children to change their speech: 'Stop! Slow down! Start again!'). In our experience, we have also been surprised at the number of adults who believe the non-fluency is a behaviour that is within children's volition. There appears to be the belief that children are deliberately speaking in an annoying way and could control themselves with extra effort or be prevented from behaving in that way by some physical punishment or threat.

◆ There is the 'do and say nothing' reaction. This is a difficult area, as one has to balance advising parents and carers not to draw children's attention to the non-fluency and, on the other hand, to acknowledge the problem. Many adults choose to ignore stammering behaviour in the belief that it is the best way to help children. In some instances, for example when children themselves are unconcerned, this may indeed be the best policy. However, when children need help in coping with their difficulties and are having problems making sense of it all, we may need to teach parents to be more supportive. Starkweather has compared the breakdown in fluency with children's breakdown in motion. If a young child falls over while out walking and has obviously hurt himself, most parents have no hesitation in going to his aid immediately and providing medical and emotional attention. When breakdown occurs in speech and the child is looking for support, the response from those adults around him may be at best tentative and considered, and at worst absent. It must be difficult for young children to understand why their parents offer support in other areas, but not in regard to speech. As clinicians, we need to help parents identify their children's need for support and acknowledgement and together consider ways of saying 'There, there. Let's kiss it better' that are appropriate to talking. We heard an excellent example of this at a bonfire. A family, consisting of Mum and Dad and three young sons were standing watching the firework display. Dad commented that the display was so impressive he wished he had remembered to bring the camera. The middle son, aged about three, asked a question about the camera but was unable to articulate the word 'camera'. He said, 'I can't say that word!' Dad's reply acknowledged his son's difficulty but was reassuringly positive: 'No, you can't, can you? But you soon will be able to.' We will consider this issue further in later chapters.

Internal demands

Self-imposed demands   A final demand we would like to propose is that of the demands that children place upon themselves: those which originate internally rather than being imposed by others or the environment. We know of children who appear to set themselves high standards of behaviour and aim to achieve goals that may be unrealistic when matched against their developmental level. At times it is apparent they have actually internalised issues that were of importance to their parents, such as the seven-year-old girl who wants to be a doctor or a dentist.

In other cases there seems to be no identifiable source for the high aspirations. One child with expressive language abilities commensurate with his chronological age showed genuine frustration at his inability to pronounce certain words which were long and contained complex sequences of consonants. In other cases, the demands may be related to confidence when taking on a performing role or in the face of odds that would reduce Superman to tears, such as performing at a school assembly when feeling under the weather.

We need to be aware of internal factors operating within the child's personality when we see him in clinic or in other circumstances. We would be alert to a number of issues, including the following:

◆ Disliking mess
◆ Poor at coping with learning new tasks or skills
◆ Wanting to get things right from the start
◆ Poor risk taking
◆ Poor tolerance of errors in themselves and others
◆ Fearing the implications of getting things wrong
◆ Expecting to do well without the necessary aptitude, practice or maturity.

It is easy to see how these factors might be transferred to bumpy speech, with negative consequences.

Developments of the Demands and Capacities Model

In 1990, Adams attempted to give more 'flesh' to the demands and capacities model and expanded the theoretical basis by posing several interesting questions:

1 If we accept that non-fluent speech hinges on the imbalance between demands and capacities, at what point does the difference become significant? Or, to put it more succinctly, what difference makes the difference? Adams argued that the capacities hold the key. He stated that even modest demands that are not far in excess of children's capacities will disrupt their fluency when their capacities have already been compromised. He suggested that cerebral insult or hereditary predisposition have such an effect on capacities. In contrast, when capacities are obviously within the normal-

superior range, it will take stringent demands which are well beyond children's capacities to produce a similar effect in their speech. It would therefore appear that, in some children, the scales are already weighted in favour of non-fluency whereas for others the weighting is in the opposite direction. It is interesting to consider children with normal-superior capacities a little more closely. If their ability to redress any imbalance is greater, we could hypothesise that it is these children who recover spontaneously. It would then follow that the children with poorer capacities are the ones who are referred to see us.

2   Let us return to the original picture of the kitchen scales to pose the second question. Does it make a difference how the scales move when there is an imbalance? Is a sudden or acute swing towards overloading the capacities and/or increasing demands more serious than an imbalance that accumulates over time in a chronic way? Adams suggested that the chances for breakdown increase significantly when demands chronically exceed capacity. We like to think that the scales may bounce back more readily when the shift is of brief duration whereas, when the imbalance is more persistent, it is harder for the capacities to counterbalance the swing. It may be that, in this instance, a pattern of 'not coping' is established. In the case of the first shift in favour of the demands, the capacities are not able to redress the balance. Because children have already experienced the effect of capacities not responding appropriately, when further weight is added to the demands the result is a greater likelihood of the negative effect being repeated.

3   The final question relates to fluency specifically. Why should it be that fluency breaks down when capacities are exceeded? Adams put forward two possible reasons:

(a) This set of demands and capacities is specific to fluent speech production. (This raises the question of whether, as maturing children develop, there are other sets of scales which can be shifted off balance to create a maladaptive response. Are there for example sets of scales for other skills such as reading? It may be too that there are different scales for different ages or stages of development.)

(b) Adams hypothesised that the precipitating factor is related to the point of development children have reached. It is at this time that fluency is the most vulnerable of all the skills which children are acquiring and therefore most at risk.

We would also suggest

(c) That the complexity of speech and language production is so great that it is one of the skills most likely to suffer at a time when children are coping with a variety of developing skills and new experiences.

(Clinicians interested in this model may like to read further. In 2000, there was an edition of the *Journal of Fluency Disorders* which contained a special section on the demands and capacities model. A number of invited papers were included and these raised some interesting points of debate.)

Strengths of the Demands and Capacities Model

In summary, we can see that this model, with our additions, has a number of strengths.

1   It allows for considerable variability in terms of presenting problems.

2   It enables us to explain stammering in terms of normality rather than abnormality. Children who stammer do not have to be deficient in terms of the capacities they possess, nor do excessive demands have to be placed upon them. The precipitating factor for non-fluency is the imbalance between the demands and capacities, and this can be enormously reassuring for both parents and children.

3   The model is especially useful when talking to parents about this complex issue. We will frequently show parents our scales model and try and apply it to their particular child, identifying what might be the capacities to be strengthened and the demands to be reduced. It does help simplify both the process and the issues in a way that both therapist and parents/carers can understand.

Difficulties with the Demands and Capacities Model

1 Our major issue with the model is in trying to reflect the interactive nature of the demands and capacities. Sometimes it is easy for parents to view factors either on one side of the scales or on the other when, in fact, they can be on both sides at the same time. For example, advanced expressive language skills can easily be seen as a capacity in terms of children's communication as a whole, but, equally, it may be a demand for them and put pressure on their fluency if other skills (such as motor) are not at the same developmental level. Children may wish to use complex sentence structures and vocabulary in pressured situations, which could increase their dysfluency in that setting. This is sometimes a difficult concept to communicate and manage in families.

2 Living and working in a multicultural city as we both do, we are sometimes aware of how the model can appear to be tied to a middle-class, western belief system. At times it seems at odds with families of different cultures who, for example, may be grounded in the medical model and perceive us as experts who will provide them with answers. In these situations, we try to help families identify the demands or pressures in the environment and ways in which they can be managed. Sometimes this is difficult, and we are aware we need to work hard to achieve this.

SUMMARY

In this chapter we have again presented the demands and capacities model as a way of bringing together the complexity of the research and the way in which the disorder presents clinically. We have described in detail the various components of the model and recent developments in the theoetical basis, giving some of our comments on recent debates. Ways in which the model can be applied to the various stages in the development of non-fluency will be discussed in subsequent chapters, with illustrations from our clinical experience.

In this chapter we will explore the theories about how stammering may develop. We will look both at the changes which may be apparent in the nature of the overt and covert stammering symptoms and at those which can occur in children's and other people's construing of their speech. The most common picture will embrace a change from tension-free speech dysfluency in young children to a communication disorder, characterised by struggle and avoidance in young adults. However, this is, of course, far from being the only possibility. There are well-documented cases in which both overt and covert symptoms have been relatively severe shortly after onset (Van Riper, 1982; Yairi & Lewis, 1984). Similarly, there are cases in which overt features remain mild, with few or no accompanying covert behaviours into adulthood. We hope this chapter will provide a framework for clinicians to make sense of these disparate presentations.

THEORIES ON THE DEVELOPMENT OF STAMMERING IN CHILDREN

As we noted in the previous chapter, theorists such as Johnson, Bloodstein and Van Riper provided us with the foundations on which modern-day theories are built. There have been others who have attempted to explain the development of stammering. Sheehan (1970, 1975), for example, stated that there was an interaction between high parental expectations and standards of behaviour and developmental factors, coupled with too little support for children. Despite his behavioural background, Sheehan seemed to believe that stammering resulted from a genetic predisposition, limitations in a child's development, and an inability to cope with demands from the environment.

When we look at these various hypotheses about stammering in children, we are struck by the paucity of data. The work of a small number of theorists represented, until recently, a substantial part of the research carried out on the development of stammering.

Current Theories & Evidence

Ehud Yairi and his co-workers have changed the face of research into the development of dysfluency in children over the past two decades. They have carried out systematic and well-planned research and, taken as a whole, their contribution to our understanding of childhood dysfluency has been very important. Their research addressed the following key issues:

◆ The onset of stammering, and how it differs from the speech of fluent children
◆ The pattern of the development of stammering
◆ The factors which determine whether or not stammering recovers or persists beyond childhood.

We propose to summarise this research under these headings.

Onset of stammering

The key findings here are:

◆ *Greatest risk for stammering onset*: 75 per cent occurs before 3 years 5 months, with the greatest risk occurring before 3 years (Yairi & Ambrose 1992a, 1992b).

Thus the third year would appear to be very important in the development of a child's fluency.

◆ *Very high levels of dysfluency* can occur near onset. Yairi & Lewis (1984) measured levels of dysfluency close to onset and found 21.54 instances of dysfluency per 100 syllables. In addition, parents rated initial stammering as moderate-severe for 28–36 per cent of children.

While parents/carers and children themselves may be very anxious about these initial levels of dysfluency, as we will see later, severity in itself may not be an important prognostic factor.

◆ *Sudden onset of stammering* is reported by 31–36 per cent of parents (Yairi, 1983; Yairi & Ambrose, 1992b).

This appears to go against some other researchers' views that stammering develops progressively, perhaps out of normal non-fluency. Yairi and his colleagues appear to have found evidence suggesting that, at least in some children, onset is sudden and can be severe from the start.

Table 2 Parents' observations of their children's speech at the onset of stammering	
Type of dysfluency	**Percentage reported at time of onset**
Syllable repetitions	95
Word repetitions	40
Sound prolongations	36
Silent periods	23
Facial contortions	18
Disrupted breathing	18
Blocks	14

◆ *Descriptive analysis of early stammering*. Yairi and his colleagues described the observations of parents on the speech of their children close to the onset of stammering (Table 2).

In addition, Yairi found that 32 per cent of parents described the onset of stammering as consisting of simple, easy repetitions with no tension or struggle, whereas 36 per cent reported moderate-severe tension associated with stammering.

◆ *Number of iterations*.[1] Syllable or word repetitions of three to five iterations at onset of stammering were reported by 85 per cent of parents. Yairi (1981) found that non-stammering children averaged between 1.1 and 1.13 iterations per repetition – that is, slightly more than one extra repetition. In later studies, Yairi and his colleagues looked at the differences between non-stammering children and their stammering peers, and found significant differences in the mean number of iterations per repetition (Yairi & Lewis, 1984; Ambrose & Yairi, 1995) (Table 3).

Thus two or more iterations occur three times more often in early stammerers than in normally speaking children.

Yairi & Lewis (1984) reached the conclusion that the number of iterations per repetition was an issue that best differentiated non-stammering children from stammering children.

---

[1] Iteration is the number of times that a sound/syllable might be repeated within one dysfluency. For example, b-b-ball is two iterations of the sound 'b' in the production of the dysfluent word 'ball'.

Table 3 Number of iterations made by children who stammer and non-stammering controls			
	Iterations (syllable and monosyllabic words)		
	1	2 or more	
	(per cent of children)	(per cent of children)	(No per 100 syllables)
Children who stammer	67	33	3.70 per 100 syllables
Non-stammering controls	87	13	0.21 per 100 syllables

◆ *Rate of repetitions*. Throneberg & Yairi (1994) carried out a spectrographic analysis of the repetitions of 20 non-stammering and stammering pre-school children. They found significant differences in the silent intervals between the repetitions: the silent interval between the iterations was the longest element in non-stammering children, but the shortest element in the iterations of beginning stammerers.

Thus children with early stammering can be distinguished from non-stammering children as their repetitions are quicker in terms of duration. It may be this increased rate of repetitions is perceived by others as being out of the child's control.

◆ *Associated physical movements* can occur at or near onset. Yairi *et al* (1993) found that 16 children had a mean of 3.18 movements per dysfluency when videotaped within 3 months of onset of stammering. They also found that this number decreased as the frequency of the dysfluency decreased.

◆ *Clustering of dysfluencies*.[2] Hubbard & Yairi (1988) found that stammering children had more than six times as many clusters as non-stammering children and the clusters were frequently longer.

◆ *Awareness*. More than 20 per cent of parents believed that their children were aware of the problem close to its onset.

Development of stammering

There have been a number of studies plotting the development of and/or recovery from stammering. Most of the recovery was noted in the first 14 months after onset

---

[2] Clusters include several dysfluencies occurring within the same word, on adjacent words and in between word spaces either before or after a dysfluent word.

of stammering, but substantial reductions were found up to two years after onset (Yairi & Ambrose, 1992a; Yairi *et al*, 1993, 1996). 65 per cent of children recovered within the first two years, and recoveries climbed to 85 per cent by the end of the study (Yairi & Ambrose, 1992a).

This suggests that clinicians need to be plotting the progress of children on a regular basis and over time.

◆ *Pattern of recovery in the six months post onset.* Yairi *et al* (1993) studied this particular period and found that:
  – the mean total dysfluency declined from 17.41 to 9.49 per 100 syllables;
  – SLDs[3] declined from 11.99 to 4.46;
  – mean facial-head movements reduced from 3.18 to 1.91 per dysfluency;
  – mean stammering severity ratings (on a seven-point scale) fell from 4.43 to 1.99.

This seems to suggest that significant improvements can occur in these earlier months. (It may be that, as clinicians, we rarely see children in this phase of spontaneous recovery because of delays in referral time and/or parents/carers 'waiting to see'.)

◆ *Pattern of recovery in the two years post onset.* Yairi & Ambrose (1992a) followed 27 untreated stammering children for 3–12 years. In the first two years, the mean total dysfluencies reduced from 16.21 to 10.35 per 100 syllables, and the mean SLDs reduced from 10.47 to 4.80. Mean SLDs declined further to 2.72 in measurements taken after the two-year period.

◆ *The importance of SLDs.* Yairi and his colleagues found differences in the occurrence of SLDs when comparing pre-school children who stammered and their non-stammering peers. Table 4 shows the mean frequency of the various types of dysfluencies per 100 syllables in pre-school children in the two groups.

---

[3] Stammer-like dysfluencies (SLDs): short element repetition (part-word and monosyllabic word repetitions), dysrhythmic phonation and tense pauses.

Table 4 Mean frequency of dysfluencies in pre-school children		
	Dysfluencies per 100 syllables (No)	
	Children who stammered	**Children who were fluent**
SLDs		
Part-word repetitions	5.64	0.55
Single-syllable repetitions	3.24	0.79
Dysrhythmic phonations	2.42	0.08
Total	11.30	0.08
Other dysfluencies	5.70	4.48

Yairi *et al* (1993) found that SLDs represented a sensitive measure of change. They found these declined from 11.99 to 6.34 to 4.46 per 100 syllables over a 6-month period, while other types of dysfluency (interjections, phrase repetitions, revisions, incomplete phrases) remained stable.

This must be one of the most important findings of Yairi's research. The indications are that we now have a significant measure in determining early stammering. Although it must never be used in isolation, the measurement of SLDs should now be a feature of all quantitative assessments of young children's speech.

◆ *Gender issues*. Boys' dysfluency did not recover in the same timescale as girls' (Yairi *et al*, 1993). Boys took longer to recover.

Persistence & recovery of stammering in children

Persistent stammering is defined (Yairi 1996) as having continued for 36 months or more. Recovered stammerers recover within 18 months of onset or between 18 and 36 months (defined as late recovered).

Information in this section is based on the following research papers: Throneberg & Yairi, 1994; Yairi *et al*, 1996; Yairi & Ambrose, 1999; Throneberg & Yairi, 2001.

◆ Between 65 and 85 per cent of children show substantial reductions in stammering, and eventual recovery from it, especially in the first two years after onset of stammering.

Potentially, this research finding could set early referral patterns back decades, as it indicates that most children do indeed grow out of early dysfluency. However, taken with the other evidence, it makes us better equipped to determine whether children who present in our clinics are in this majority or in the 25 per cent (approximately) who are at risk.

◆ All children show an increase in the severity of their stammering soon after onset, followed by a decrease, but the persistent group shows slower changes which seem to plateau after 12 months. Other groups may continue to recover 3–4 years post onset.

◆ Gender issues. There are differences in both persistence and recovery in relation to the rate of recovery in boys and girls (Table 5).
The ratio for persistence is 3.67 (boys):1 (girls).
In relation to recovery, girls were found to recover more quickly – 12–18 months after the onset of the stammering. Boys recovered at a slower rate – 24–36 months after onset.

There appear to be significant differences in recovery related to gender. It is interesting to speculate whether these are connected to language development issues in particular, or to the accelerated rate of development generally of girls at this age.

◆ The recovered group had a higher level of SLDs, which then changed rapidly for the early recoverers and more slowly for the later recoverers.

◆ In the persistent group, the SLDs showed little change.

Again, we see in these data the importance of the measurement of SLDs over time.

◆ Descriptive differences between persistent stammering and recovered groups. Yairi and his colleagues found identifiable differences between the two groups from 7 months after onset, although the differences were more obvious after 12 months. The differences included:

Table 5 Persistence of and recovery from stammering in boys and girls		
	Boys	**Girls**
Persistence	30	18
Recovery	70	82

- Type of dysfluency (Table 6).

  In addition, the persistent group showed less decrease in disrhythmic phonations than the recovered group. The rate of repetitions was also different in that the persistent group showed slightly shorter pause times than the recovered group, and the latter group gradually slowed the rate of repetitions as they recovered.

- The group in whom dysfluency persisted were older at onset by nearly 11 months.

- Children in the persistent group had a greater number of relatives who stammered into adulthood; thus persistence seems to be genetic.

Developmental Dimensions

Yairi (1997) put forward a way of considering the various facets of the development of stammering. He described four dimensions, which he believed can distinguish the dysfluent speech of early childhood stammering.

1 *Quantitative*. The measurement of frequency of dysfluency, the number of iterations in repetitions, and the duration of the dysfluency.

2 *Qualitative*. Different types of dysfluencies (SLDs or other dysfluencies), clustering of dysfluencies.

3 *Physical*. Temporal characteristics, rate of repetitions.

4 *Physiological*. Associated behaviours (head and neck movements), tension.

While we agree that these dimensions are important and are essential to any clinical assessment, we also suggest that there is a fifth dimension of equal import, which Yairi has not included.

Table 6 Differences in types of dysfluency between children who recovered and those who persisted in stammering		
	SLDs (%)	Other dysfluencies (%)
Persistent group	.66	.34
Recovered group	.24	.76

5 *Psychological.*

It is our assertion that it is this psychological dimension that may account for several features in the development of stammering for a number of children in this age group. For example, some children appear to move from repeating whole words to part-word (sound or syllable) repetitions. This fragmentation of language may be triggered by a psychological process that stems from a belief in the child that the repetitions are unacceptable and need to be changed in some way/brought under control. Similarly, the move from easy dysfluencies to tense blocks with struggle and associated physical behaviours may be another reaction sparked off in the same way.

We also believe that further changes can be wrought in the development of the stammer which send the overt features 'underground', and as a result the stammer becomes more covert and deep rooted. This is a serious development, which is not totally accounted for in Yairi's other four dimensions.

The final section of this chapter will consider this fifth dimension in more detail. We will describe its importance and outline the factors to be considered by clinicians.

PSYCHOLOGICAL ISSUES: THE FIFTH DIMENSION

In this section we will look at the psychological dimension in terms of the various hypotheses that have been put forward as to why children change their pattern of stammering. We are also aware that there are some children whose pattern of dysfluency remains relatively unchanged from onset. This does not mean that their constructions about dysfluency will also remain constant. (Our understanding of children's psychological development would suggest that this aspect of development is as dynamic a process as any other.) So we assert that this dimension may well have applications to children, whether or not their speech is subject to different patterns.

Change from 'Stammering' to 'Stammerer'

Hayhow (1992) proposed that looking at the development of what we have called 'the fifth dimension' involves exploring the movement from 'stammering' to 'stammerer'.

Some authorities suggest that this change will be gradual and not associated with any specific stressful event (Van Riper, 1982; Starkweather, 1987; Peters & Guitar, 1991). They argue that it starts with a child's fleeting awareness that their speech may be problematic. If we accept this view, then we might speculate as to how children may start to become aware that their speech is different in some way. There could be internal and external responses to dysfluency that influence this process. Internal responses are those within children – perhaps a moment of consternation or frustration at not being able to say a word at exactly at the time they want to, or a sensation of 'stuckness' in trying to produce the word. External responses are those of others, often very subtle, which may give children clues that something is not quite right or acceptable. The listener may change his expression, momentarily lose eye contact, tense during and relax after the moment of stammering or give an instruction to 'slow down'. Children may begin with an awareness that is confined only to the moment of stammering and is not present on every dysfluent utterance; there is little concern and no anticipation of difficulty, the 'problem' is purely one of speech and has no other implications for them. The development of this dimension sees a change in terms of an awareness that speech is 'not quite right'. This, in time, can lead some children to try to alter their speech by changing some of the other dimensions to which Yairi refers: the type of dysfluency, the number of interations in the repetitions, the duration of the dysfluency, and/or the degree of effort they put into speaking. In addition, other 'demands' – both internal and external – may outweigh the 'capacities' that children use to deal with them (see Chapter 2).

Altered Construing

Hayhow (1992) suggests that not only may children then try to change dimensions related to their behaviour (first order change), but, as they begin to feel a loss of both physical and psychological control when stammering, they may also alter the way in which they think about the 'problem' (second order change) (Watzlawick *et al*, 1974). They will try to make sense of their dysfluency as best they can. The way in which they do this can narrow their options. They may start to construe their world in a restricted way in terms of 'how it is for speaking in'. For example, children may construe themselves in different situations as fluent/not fluent and may construe others in terms of being easy to talk to/difficult to talk to. In so doing, they seek to bring about some order and predictability to a problem which they cannot otherwise understand.

Providing Solutions

In addition, Hayhow (1992) proposed that stammering may begin to provide solutions to other problems that children encounter. It might, for example, serve as a way for non-assertive children to gain the attention of listeners. It may ensure an escape from challenging school tasks or provide a legitimate reason for a difficulty in making friends. This point has been developed by Perkins (1992, p120) who described these solutions in terms of 'pay-offs', which, he argued, can become addictive and in time lead children to build their lives around the concept 'I am a stutterer'.

Parents' Construing of Stammering

Understanding the development of children's stammering also necessitates understanding the meaning it has been given by parents. These important people in the lives of children will also be attempting to make sense of the problem, and may experiment with many different ways of trying to change the child's behaviour. The solutions which they have attempted may, however, have served to maintain and develop the problem. Hayhow (1992) pointed out how failure to achieve change can be very invalidating for parents, and lead them to negatively construe the child who stammers in other aspects in addition to fluency. Stammering may also serve a specific role in a troubled family.

Parental Behaviours

In looking at parents' responses, Starkweather (1987, p145) stated that 'people respond most to the behaviour of other people'. This seems to us to be a very important point to consider, for two main reasons. First, it helps us to understand some of the behaviours that parents demonstrate (such as increased speech rate, interruptions) as being a reaction to, but not a cause of, the dysfluency. Secondly, we can convey this information to the parents. In our experience this often helps to reduce the guilt felt by many parents, and to alter their belief that the stammer must have been caused by something they have done. It may also help them experiment with new and more positive ways of responding.

The Child's Attitude to Stammering

Starkweather (1987) suggested that the process by which children develop particular attitudes towards stammering is much the same as the process by which they develop their attitude to anything else. He gives the example of a child who develops a fear of dogs or a delight in music because of a similar attitude in a parent. He notes how parents' verbal and/or non-verbal responses to dysfluency may indicate discomfort or hurt, which in turn can influence children's attitudes in a similar way.

The Communication Environment

Starkweather (1987) also saw the development of stammering as being linked to the communicative environment. He explained the changes that sometimes take place in children's speech as being dependent on specific environmental factors, and gave some interesting examples as to how speech may be affected. If the child experiences time pressure, Starkweather suggests that the child may try to shorten the elements that he repeats – a typical scenario might be a shift from whole-word to part-word repetitions. If, for whatever reason, there is pressure on the child to produce more complex language than his motor system can accommodate, Starkweather believes that the dysfluencies may become hesitant, with discontinuities occurring at particular places such as clause boundaries or before infrequently used words. Similarly, he suggests that negative reactions produce more effort and hence struggle and avoidance, whereas demand speech, which induces cognitive pressure, may produce discontinuities as a result. Although these ideas do not appear to be backed up by the more recent research findings by Yairi and others, they do appear to be logical and have an intuitive appeal. Should it be possible to make empirical links between specific environmental pressures and specific types of dysfluency, we might become more confident in suggesting specific interventions.

Development of Tension

Following on from some of the easier dysfluencies mentioned above, Starkweather (1987, p148) saw the next developmental stage as typically involving tension at a laryngeal level. He gave three examples of how these are realised in speech. The first is 'prolonged vowels with pitch rise'. The second involves 'broken words' (vowel is initiated, cut off by cord closure and then re-started). The third, 'increased loudness', can occur in conjunction with repetitions of vowels or may continue over whole utterances. Starkweather argued that this stage is followed by struggle behaviour, which may be initiated at various points in the body and used in order to force sounds out. The tension involved is often visible, particularly in the face and neck.

Use of Starters

As the struggle behaviour intensifies, children begin to get stuck and when they try to initiate sound, there are times when none comes. Starkweather proposed that this is the point at which the use of 'starters' begins. These can involve particular parts of the body, such as leg stamping or head moving. They may involve the use of 'easy' words as a means of access to more difficult ones, or increased use of 'ums' and 'ers'. Sometimes the starters come from the suggestions of others to 'start again' or 'take a deep breath'. Generally, the devices work well initially and help children to launch their speech quite successfully. However, usually the potency of the strategy decreases, but it may still persist as a habit and become part of the stammering behaviour, no longer serving any useful purpose.

Avoidance Behaviours

It is clear to us that the development of avoidance behaviours is part of the psychological dimension of stammering in children. These often appear as children get older and are one of the more sophisticated devices they use to hide their stammer. We see a range of avoidance behaviours in children used in a variety of ways to manage the communicative challenges children face. Changing words, non-participation, circumlocution, distractions (coughing, dropping something), pretending to forget, faking lack of interest, are just some of the methods we have encountered in children who are trying to prevent others from realising the extent of their problem. A 13-year-old boy managed to keep his quite severe stammer completely hidden from his teachers most successfully, by carefully scanning what he might say in answer to a question before deciding whether to reply or to pretend he did not know the answer. He was able to answer enough questions and to initiate enough conversations in all school situations not to be perceived as having any speech problem.

By the time children are using avoidance as a way of coping, it is likely that their journey from stammering to stammerer is complete. They are now construing themselves in speaking situations in terms of fluency and other people in terms of the effect on their speech. The environment may well continue to change to accommodate a child's 'differentness'; for example, they may not be expected to read in class or to take on responsibilities that involve speaking, which further reinforces the 'usefulness' of the avoidance strategy.

SUMMARY

As a conclusion to this chapter, we will summarise what we believe to be the important issues in the development of stammering in children. Taken as a whole, recent studies have major clinical implications for those of us who are faced with parents and children on a daily basis asking the question, 'Is this stammering?' While we still have no definitive crystal ball, we now have a number of factors that can help us decide which children need intervention and at what stage it is going to be of most use. The following summary of risk factors (Table 7) attempts to include the qualitative and quantitative information we now have available, in addition to our own observations of clients.

Table 7 Summary of risk factors for the development of stammering

◆ *SLDs* – presence and persistence of these types of dysfluencies are significant

◆ *Rate of repetitions* – faster rate is of more concern

◆ *Change* – look at pattern of change since onset. No change is of concern. Slower change is better than none at all

◆ *Length of time child has been dysfluent* – if longer than 12 months, the child is more at risk

◆ *Genetics* – not just having a family member who stammers, but looking at the occurrence of persistent stammering in the family

◆ *Gender* – boys more at risk than girls. NB: girls who are not recovering should be looked at carefully

◆ *Psychological change* – evidence that children are reconstruing their dysfluencies in ways that compromise their communication. Evidence that children are reconstruing themselves in ways that compromise the individuals they are and hope to be.

In approaching the assessment of stammering, we agree with the rationale offered by Crowe *et al* (2000, p1) that 'assessment and treatment should address as many of the effects of stuttering on the client's communicative behaviour and living status as possible'. Our adherence to a view of stammering as multifactorial means that we need to address its varying components in our assessment and be mindful in reassessment, that any or all of the factors may change over time. If stammering is a multifactorial problem, we will need a multifactorial evaluation which 'will result in a composite of interactive factors which reflects an individual's communicative behaviour at any given time' (Susca & Healey, 2000). We also need to ensure that our assessment is comprehensive by taking into account all Yairi's (1997) four dimensions as well as our own fifth dimension.

An important point for British speech & language therapists when thinking about assessment is that the Royal College of Speech and Language Therapists now has a set of clinical guidelines for disorders of fluency. These include the imperative to use published scales where possible and the need to include measures of the child's dysfluency and reactions to it, so that representative speech samples can be obtained.

When carrying out an assessment (and indeed treatment) with children and their parents/carers we need also to be aware of the cultural background from which they come. Hall (2000) states that in order to be culturally competent a clinician needs to be aware of issues related to culture, race, gender, sexual orientation, and social class. Verbal and non-verbal styles may vary a great deal between cultures. Many published assessments tend to be monocultural, for example, scoring negatively for reduced eye contact, when in some cultures direct eye contact would be seen as a taboo in some circumstances. Different cultures also view stammering very differently, and it is important for the clinician to be familiar with these differences. Manning (2001) addressed this point in his assessment battery through a 'cultural factors' assessment sheet, which is given to the child's carer to complete. This contains questions under the headings of cultural identity, assimilation, environment, attitudes and beliefs. Clinicians may not wish to use the form as it is presented, but may find some of the questions it asks helpful in prompting them as to issues they may need to address.

OVERT FEATURES

In Chapter 5 we will look at features of early stammering and how these are qualitatively and quantitatively different from those of normal non-fluency. In this chapter, we look at practical ways of assessing these features. In addition, we discuss ways of assessing dysfluency in children in whom such a diagnosis is clear and the assessment is to be used for ascertaining severity and/or as a base measure against which to reassess in the future.

The Speech Sample

By listening to a child talking informally, it is certainly possible to note down various observations about the nature, type, duration and so on of the dysfluencies. However, in order to describe a child's dysfluencies fully and accurately, an audio- or video-recorded sample should be taken. Many clinicians suggest that different types of speaking tasks should be addressed, in order to assess overall severity. A child who stammers on an 'easier' task, such as rote speaking or naming, may well be deemed to have a more severe problem. Rustin (1987) suggested that the following areas should be assessed:

- Automatic speech
- Echoic speech
- Reading
- Naming pictures
- Monologue
- Questions
- Conversation, including normal stressors, such as questions and interruptions.

Because of the dynamic nature of stammering, some of the behaviours the child exhibits may not be apparent when the assessment is taking place. Manning (2001, p187) suggested that, if this is the case, the clinician should make attempts to elicit the behaviours by 'creating a speaking situation where, temporarily at least, the demands on the child exceed his ability to use his speech production system'. As examples of the ways in which this can be done, he suggested the following:

- Indicating a loss of attention, for example, by turning away from the child as he talks
- Asking the child for rapid responses to a number of questions
- Asking abstract or difficult-to-answer questions
- Asking the child to read at a level above his ability range
- Asking the child to describe pictures, at a rate at which he is unable to finish one response before another is demanded
- Interrupting the child
- Using additional listeners.

Manning pointed out the need to explain the purpose of such procedures to the parents, and for the clinician to use as few of these types of activities as are necessary to elicit the desired behaviours in the child.

By making a recording, the clinician can take time to make an accurate appraisal of the various features of the child's dysfluency. It is generally agreed that a sample of between 300 and 500 syllables is needed. Because of the problem of variability of a child's stammering, Yairi (1997) suggested that speech samples of 500 syllables be taken on two separate occasions.

The setting for recording the sample

Manning also suggested that assessments are made in different settings than the clinic, in order to get the most realistic picture of the child. He advocated the home or school setting as being more natural, although we would think that the logistics of recording a child at school would make such a venture undesirable. Asking the parents to make a video- or audiotape recording of the child is another possibility. We have found this to be very helpful, especially when the child is more fluent in the clinic. Parents may feel they are not believed by the clinician when they say that their child's stammering is much more severe than has been demonstrated in the clinical setting; providing a tape gives them the opportunity to be sure that this is not the case.

The analysis of the sample

The recording of 500 syllables of a child's speech is not in itself a time-consuming activity. Analysing the recording may be a different matter. However, we would suggest that such an exercise is not only good practice but can help 'tune in' a clinician's ear to important things for which to listen.

Analysing a speech sample is far from easy. When we have given groups of clinicians such an exercise, we have had as many analyses as we had clinicians, and in addition we two authors often hear the same tape very differently. This, of course, begs the question of whether the task is therefore worthwhile. We would argue that anything that helps us to listen more carefully to what is actually going on when we hear a child stammering can only be useful. For assessment purposes, it is intra-rater reliability rather than inter-rater reliability that concerns us. In other words, we need only be consistent with ourselves, unless we are undertaking research in which an agreed level of inter-rater reliability is essential.

There are many coding systems now in use on both sides of the Atlantic. Our personal preference is that used as part of the Codes for the Human Analysis of Transcripts system (CHAT) (Berstein-Ratner *et al*, 1996) and we would recommend that clinicians read the appropriate reference for a full description, as we can only provide a summary here (Table 8).

Dysfluencies

Types of dysfluency – qualitative dimensions

Most writers on dysfluency propose that analysing the type of dysfluency in a child's speech gives an indication of risk (Yairi & Lewis, 1984; Conture, 1997; Shapiro, 1999).

In listening to this area of a child's dysfluency, we are looking both for more normal dysfluencies and for those which are thought to differentiate normal non-fluency from developing stuttering. The following types of dysfluencies (which are listed

Table 8 Summary of dysfluency coding (CHAT)

Type of Dysfluency	Example	Code
*SLDs**		
i. Sound/syllable repetition	ba-ba-by	ba(&1be)by
	th-th-th-that	th(&3th)at
ii. Whole-word repetition	that's that's that's interesting	that's (/2) interesting
iii. Prolongations	ssssomething	s:omething
	soooomething	so:mething
iv. Blocks	^I tend to have blocks	^I tend to have blocks
v. Broken words	Is that a rhin......oceros?	Is that a rhin~oceros?
Normal Dysfluencies		
i. Hesitations (unfilled pauses)	I can meet you in 20mins	I can meet you in # 20mins
ii. Filled pauses	Well, how are you?	Well@fp how are you?
	My name, you know, is Trudy	My name you+knowfp is Trudy
iii. Phrase repetitions	I'm going to	I'm going to
	I'm going to town	I'm+going+to@pr town

* SLD: stammer/stutter-like dysfluency

here in approximate order of being typical (that is, more normal) to atypical (less normal/stammering-like dysfluencies [SLDs]) should therefore be noted:

◆ Hesitations/unfilled pauses

◆ Interjections

◆ Phrase repetitions/revisions

◆ Filled pauses/fillers

◆ Word repetitions

◆ Sound repetitions

◆ Part-word/syllable repetitions

◆ Broken words

◆ Prolongations

◆ Blocks.

To measure types of dysfluencies Use taped, transcribed analysis to record the numbers of each type of dysfluency heard on each syllable and to present them as a percentage of total dysfluency and/or syllables spoken (using the formula given below for frequency).

Frequency of dysfluency – quantitative dimensions

In assessing the frequency of a child's dysfluencies, we are looking at two areas.

1 *The total amount of dysfluency of any sort.* Curlee (1999, p10) stated that 'if a child's percentage of total dysfluencies exceeds 10 per cent of the words or syllables uttered, I believe the child is at risk for a fluency disorder'. Studies suggest, in addition to this finding, that children who stammer are at least twice as dysfluent as those who do not (Zebrowski, 1995).

How to score total dysfluency Use the following equation:

$$\textbf{percentage syllables stammered} = \frac{\text{total no of dysfluencies (counted on each syllable)}}{\text{total syllables spoken}} \times 100$$

2 *The frequency of different sorts of dysfluency.* The presence of 3 per cent or more SLDs is generally believed to be indicative of stammering (Yairi, 1997; Curlee, 1999). SLDs comprise part-word and monosyllabic word repetitions, dysrhythmic phonation (including prolongations), and tense pauses. All can occur in the speech of non-stammering children, but occur far more in children who stammer. (This is also considered significant in terms of severity, as will be outlined below.)

How to measure frequency of dysfluencies Apply the equation:

$$\textbf{percentage SLDs} = \frac{\text{total no of SLDs}}{\text{total syllables spoken}} \times 100$$

Riley's Stuttering Severity Instrument (1994) converts the percentage dysfluency into a 'task score' which, together with task scores for duration and physical concomitants, produces a five-point total severity score ranging from very mild to very severe.

Crowe *et al* (2000) suggested recording the results for both total dysfluency and each type of dysfluency using scales of 1–6 (from 1 = 0–2 per cent frequency to 6 = more than 30 per cent). Following such an approach would, we suggest, enable the clinician to note changes in both total frequency and – perhaps more significantly – type of dysfluency, which may be important prognostically.

Duration of dysfluency – physical dimensions

Shapiro (1999, p14) referred to duration as 'the temporal length, usually in seconds for clinical purposes, of an instance of stuttering, often averaged over a randomly selected sample of several instances of stuttering within a speaking context'. The body of evidence regarding the significance of duration of dysfluencies is limited and inconsistent (Yairi, 1997). Yairi advised that such measures cannot currently be used to differentiate stammering from normal childhood dysfluency. Conture (1997) believed measurement of duration to be useful in describing the quality of dysfluency, as opposed to measures of frequency, which describe its quantity. He saw it as a reasonable clinical perspective that, the longer the duration, the more severe the stammering. Crowe *et al* (2000) included a protocol for measuring duration of dysfluencies (shown below) that is similar to that suggested by Conture. Crowe *et al* suggested using this as part of assessment and prognosis, and also as an outcome tool in terms of the effect therapy has in increasing communication effectiveness and reducing handicap.

To measure duration of dysfluencies Using a recorded sample (as suggested above), Crowe *et al* (2000) suggested selecting a sample of 10 consecutive dysfluencies (or fewer if there are not 10 in the sample) to be timed using a stopwatch. These can then be used to calculate the mean, standard deviation, range, mode and median. Crowe's group also suggested that the clinician should note any particularly long dysfluencies, but should not include these in any of the calculations.

Duration is also used in Riley's Stuttering Severity Instrument (SSI-3) (1994). This computes the average duration of the three longest stammering events (from 'fleeting' to '1 minute') and converts these to a task score (see 'Frequency of dysfluency' above).

Differentiating & rating severity of stammering

Severity is currently measured as a function of several dimensions: frequency, duration and type. Ambrose & Yairi (1999) have formalised this by using a calculation that weights the 'stammer-like disfluencies' and differentiates them from 'other dysfluencies', which they regard as more typical of normally dysfluent speech. 'Not only quantity, but the proportion, extent and duration of disfluencies distinguish stuttering from normally dysfluent speech' (p905).

How to calculate severity of stammering The following equation is used:

Severity = [(PWR + SSWR per 100 syllables) × ru] + (2 × DP per 100 syllables)

where PWR = part-word repetition, SSWR = single-syllable word repetition, ru = mean number of iterations, and DP = dysrhythmic phonation

Secondary Symptoms – Physiological Dimensions

Secondary behaviours are significant because they show us that children are reacting in some way to their stammering, by trying to do something to stop it from happening or to 'force' the words out. Shapiro (1999) divided secondary characteristics into two types, non-speech (for example, face and body movements and tension) and speech (for example, pitch rises, laryngeal tension, audible inhalations or exhalations). Crowe *et al* (2000) believe that these behaviours should form part of any assessment, because they are likely to make stuttering look unnatural and thus be more handicapping to the person who stammers. As will be discussed below, Riley (1994) used secondary symptoms as a measure of severity of stammering.

To measure secondary symptoms

Crowe *et al* (2000) devised an assessment form which describes six facial behaviours and six body movements (with space for two additional unspecified ones of each) and scored them on a scale of 0 (= never) to 6 (= consistent in all speech). These are then collated, first on to two overall ratings (face and body) of accompanying physical behaviours scales, and finally on to a scale entitled 'overall rating of accompanying physical behaviours'. These last three scales are rated from

0 (unnoticeable) to 6 (potentially handicapping). Crowe *et al*'s scales do not include secondary speech characteristics.

Riley's (1994) Stuttering Severity Instrument 3 rates physical concomitants in four areas (distracting sounds, facial grimaces, head movements and movements of the extremities) on a scale of 0–5. This produces a third 'task score', which is used, together with scores for frequency and duration, to rate stammering severity.

Other Overt Characteristics

Rate of speech

Having a measure of a child's speaking rate may be useful in helping the clinician decide if rate control should be a part of any treatment package. A child's speech when stammering, especially if the duration of individual stammers is particularly long, may of course appear very slow. If this were the case, a desired therapy aim would be an overall faster speaking rate. However, fast-speaking children who tend to repeat syllables rather than block will reflect this in faster than average syllable-per-minute scores. For these children, whose speaking rates may put too much pressure on the rest of their speech system, it is likely that a decrease in speech rate will be a desired outcome of therapy.

It can be useful to compare measures of speaking rates in reading and in conversational speech. Often a child who avoids words will have a higher conversational rate in syllables per second than on the same measure in reading, where avoidance strategies are more difficult to use.

To measure rate of speech The rate of speech is calculated as:

$$\text{Syllables per minute} = \frac{\text{Syllables read or spoken}}{\text{Time taken in seconds}} \times 60$$

These measurements need to be compared with average speaking rates in non-stammering children. Shapiro (1999) quotes a number of studies of the speaking rates of non-stammering American children. We have been unable to find comparable figures for British children, and so cannot say how accurate the American figures are for this population. These studies include:

- Peters & Guitar (1991) – norms for children aged 6, 8, 10 and 12 years respectively are 140–175, 150–180, 165–215 and 165–220 syllables per minute (spm).
- Kelly & Conture (1992) – norms for boys aged from 3 years 2 months to 4 years 10 months (average age 4 years 0 months) are 177.6 spm.
- Ryan (1992) – for children of 2 years 10 months to 5 years 9 months (mean 4 years 5 months) the average rate for boys was 164.1 spm and for girls 176.3 spm.

Place/location of dysfluency

Place of dysfluency is mentioned very little in the literature, other than as a descriptor of stammering. Shapiro (1999) noted, for example, that stammering in children occurs more often at the beginning of sentences and on conjunctions and pronouns than in nouns and interjections, making the point that language and stammering affect each other. Crowe *et al* (2000) argued that collecting information about the location of dysfluencies is helpful, for two reasons. They suggested that knowing where dysfluencies occur is helpful therapeutically in terms of the use of control techniques. In addition, they believe that it can be useful in differential diagnosis of developmental and acquired stammering – in the former the dysfluencies are most likely to occur on the initial phoneme, and in the latter they can occur in all positions.

To measure location of dysfluencies The protocol proposed by Crowe *et al* (2000) uses the transcribed, recorded sample and counts the dysfluencies that occurred on initial syllables and those which occurred on all other syllables. Each is calculated as a percentage.

Consistency

Crowe *et al* (2000) further suggested that subjective parental ratings of consistency should be undertaken, in terms of both frequency and type of stuttering. They cite

Bloodstein (1995), indicating that greater consistency is suggestive of greater severity or more advanced stuttering. Crowe *et al* also suggested that such a measurement can help with prognosis – the less consistent the stuttering, the better the prognosis. In addition, this measure can help in a differential diagnosis between acquired and developmental stuttering (the former being more consistent).

Naturalness

Crowe *et al* (2000) included a measure of communicative naturalness, to be completed by the clinician and containing the following measures:

◆ Rate and flow of speech
◆ Vocal and voice quality
◆ Vocal range
◆ Pitch
◆ Mean latency and duration of response
◆ Intelligibility
◆ Circumlocution
◆ Substitution
◆ Revision
◆ Accompanying physical behaviours
◆ Comfort level of speech.

These are averaged to produce a six-point 'overall naturalness of speech' measure on a scale from 0 (completely natural) to 6 (potentially handicapping).

Other

Shapiro (1999) included a section in his assessment protocols that he called 'other'. Of those we have not already discussed, he included the following:

◆ Tempo
◆ Regularity
◆ Relative tension
◆ Smoothness of transitions.

He gave no suggestions as to how these might be measured, but we would suggest that they are noted by the clinician if they appear to be unusual/significant.

COVERT FEATURES – PSYCHOLOGICAL DIMENSION

It is important not to assume that, because a child does not verbally express negative emotions or show any signs of avoidance, he is unaware of any difficulty in talking. In young children, awareness is often fleeting, associated with a particular moment of stammering. Awareness may not be associated with severity; it may be related more to the degree of the child's need to put over their point at a given moment in time. Awareness may be apparent at some times and absent at others. If a child is showing signs of struggle in speaking, it is very likely he also has some awareness of the difficulty. Struggle is, after all, a way of trying to change what is happening, and to gain some control.

Assessment of Emotions Connected with Stammering

Informal assessment

Ask the client George Kelly, the father of Personal Construct Psychology, is often quoted as saying that if we want to know what is wrong with someone, we should ask them. This holds true not only for our adult clients, but also for the children we see. Their answers can provide us with useful insight into how they perceive any difficulty, whether it is something which is discussed with them at home and, if so, how it is discussed. Clearly, the way we talk to children about their dysfluency varies according to their age and developmental stage. Sometimes it is easier to ask children while they are doing something, maybe drawing a picture or playing a game. With many children we may simply ask 'why has your Mum/Dad brought you here to see me?' Older children typically give an answer like 'because I stammer', but some will say 'I don't know' or look at a parent for help. If the child's response is 'don't know', the clinician may prompt by telling them a little about our job with people who sometimes find talking difficult and asking if that is ever the case for them.

Children's answers often amaze the clinician, the parent, or both. We have had 'because I stammer/stutter' as a response from very young children whose parents tell us they have never used such a word in the child's presence. Similarly, we are often told 'I can't talk'. Others tell us they have come to play or 'to see the doctor'. Some very young children have made us surprised at how articulately they are able to describe their bumpy speech.

Asking children about home and school not only is a way of learning about the sort of people they are, but also can give us clues as to how the stammer may affect them, and how supported they feel. Clearly the nature of the questions will vary according to the child's age, and with older children questions will be very direct ('Do you answer questions in class?', 'What do your parents say when you stammer?', 'Are you teased about your stammering?').

When we have ascertained that children have some awareness about their stammering. we can ask them more specific questions about it.

Draw an iceberg (Sheehan, 1958): From about 9 years, children can understand the iceberg concept of stammering and are capable of discussing and drawing their own. This exercise is a useful one to share with parents, who can sometimes be surprised at the level of negative emotions and avoidance behaviours the child articulates in this way. As prompts for the iceberg with older children, avoidance and negative emotions checklists (Turnbull & Stewart, 1999) can be used, either as they stand or adapted by the clinician to make them more simple/straightforward.

Draw/describe the stammer Often it is hard for children to respond verbally to direct questions about stammering, but easier when they can use a different form to do so. Giving children free range with pencils, chalk, felt-tip pens and collage materials to 'show me what your stammer looks like' can often be a freeing experience for children for whom verbal expression may be fraught with problems. Another useful technique is to ask more 'lateral thinking'-type questions. Examples of such questions could be, 'If your stammer was an animal what sort of animal would it be?', 'If you gave your stammer a name what would you call it?', 'What colour is your stammer?' and 'What does your stammer eat for breakfast?' Children are far more used than adults to using their imaginations, and the clinician may find it easier to engage with children at this level.

Draw on your Emotions (Sunderland & Engleheart, 1993) This resource book is subtitled *'Creative Ways to Explore, Express and Understand Important Feelings'*. The book uses pictures and images to help people do this. It contains sections headed 'Your life', 'Who are you?', 'Your feelings', 'Things which make your life difficult', 'The good things in life', 'Feelings about places', and 'Feelings about other people'. The contents are described as relevant and adaptable for anyone aged 6 years and upwards. We find the book useful for clients who may find words inadequate, unhelpful or too difficult to express aloud. It can be particularly helpful for clients with very severe overt stammers who take a long while to say anything and find the effort of trying to explain something emotional too exhausting to attempt. The book is written with an adult audience in mind, but sections are certainly suitable for older children and adolescents.

Scaling We have found scaling to be a very useful technique to use with older children as well as with adults. Developed by the Brief Therapy Training Center in Milwaukee, this is a tried and tested Solution Focused Brief Therapy Technique (de Shazer, 1991). The standard scale is 1–10 but it can be any number that seems appropriate. Words can also be used and the scale can be made bigger or smaller (for example, answers to a question such as 'How much do you avoid reading out in class?' could be on a scale such as 'all the time, most of the time, a lot, quite a lot, a little, not at all', or 'always, sometimes, never'). Scales can be used in as many ways as the clinician's inventiveness allows. In terms of covert stammering, scales can be used to measure avoidance, emotions, and degree of perceived handicap, in addition to other areas such as motivation, change, severity, aims and expectations. The list is endless. We find a 'botheredness' scale particularly useful, both as an initial measure and then to look at change which has occurred. We ask, 'on a scale of 1–10, where 10 means you think about your stammering all the time, you wake up thinking of it, you go to bed thinking of it and you think of it all the rest of the time too, and 1 means you never give it a thought, where are you now?'

Sentence completion One of the methods we use to find out about the child's view of themselves is through sentence completion. We supply the first few words of a sentence for the child to complete. Sometimes stammering is mentioned in the answers, sometimes it is not. Often the answers give us a sense of the child's construing of self. The types of statements we make are:

- My Mum/Dad/teacher/sister/brother thinks I am ...
- My Mum/Dad/teacher/sister/brother thinks I am good at/not good at ...
- I think I am ...
- I think I am good at/not good at ...
- If I had three wishes they would be ...
- A good thing about school/friends/brothers/parents is ...
- A bad thing about school/friends/brothers/parents is ...
- My stammer is ...
- When I stammer I ...

Personal construct psychology techniques In Chapter 7 ('Confirmed Stammering'), a range of techniques taken from personal construct psychology is described. These can be adapted for use in assessing children of different ages and stages of stammering development.

Tree people (Wilson, 1988) Many clinicians will be familiar with this picture of a tree with amorphous figures standing on or near it, some together, some alone, some active, others still. We use it as a way of exploring a child's construing in a non-threatening way. We can ask questions about the child: 'Which one is most/least like you?'; 'Which one would you like/not like to be?' We may ask about significant others ('Which one could be your Dad/Mum/brother/sister/friend?'). We also sometimes ask about which picture represents the child when he stammers or his speech is 'bumpy' or when his speaking is smooth. We have found varying levels of response – there are some children who want to tell us who almost everyone is on the picture, some need prompts to name anyone, some express some important and revealing facts, ideas and feelings ('that's me because I am often on my own in the playground'), others are very concrete in their descriptions ('that's my brother because he likes climbing trees').

Formal Assessments

In this section, we give details of a number of assessments that we have found to be useful. In addition, we name some others which are available. It is for clinicians to judge which, if any, of these are suitable for their own particular situation. Clearly, to complete the whole battery of assessments would be overwhelming for a child, as well as extremely time consuming for all involved.

Attitudes towards stammering

Three notable methods of assessment have been published.

◆ *The A19 scale* (Andre & Guitar, 1979) contains 19 questions that demand a yes or no response from the child to questions such as, 'Is it hard to talk to your teachers?', 'Are you a little afraid to talk on the phone?'. Scores are worked out by allocating a point to the response that is deemed to be more likely in a child who stammers. A higher score suggests more negative attitudes towards stammering. We find some of the questions quite confusing for children. An example is, 'If you did not know a person, would you tell them your name?'. In an age where children are taught not to talk to strangers, we find ourselves trying to rephrase this in a more acceptable way, such as '... if your Mum or Dad thought it was OK to talk to them'! Other questions, such as 'Are you sometimes unhappy?' or 'Are you upset when someone interrupts you?' would seem to be likely to get the 'yes' vote from many children, with a stammer or without. However, the assessment is quick and easy to administer, and norms are given for stammering and non-stammering children. Therefore, despite some of our misgivings, we see it as a useful part of our assessments.

◆ *Attitudes Towards Stuttering* (Crowe *et al*, 2000). This assessment contains 20 statements to which the child can respond 'agree' or 'disagree'. The assessment is not scored, and Crowe *et al* state its aims as being to initiate discussion of attitudes. There is no clear-cut appropriate preferable response to some of the statements (for example, 'ignoring a person when he or she stutters is a good idea'; 'it is normal to feel somewhat embarrassed when one stutters in public').

◆ *The Communication Attitude Test – revised (CAT-R)* (De Nil & Brutten, 1991) also contains statements which, this time, the child responds to with 'true' or 'false'. Some of the wording needs to be changed for British clinicians (for example, 'it is harder for me to give a report in class than it is for the other kids'). Many of the statements are similar, presumably to check for consistency of responses (for example, 'I don't talk right', 'I like the way I talk', 'I am not a good talker'). Points are given for each response that matches the one in the key. Averages are given for stammering and non-stammering children.

Emotions about Stammering

◆ *Emotional responses to stuttering* (Crowe *et al*, 2000). Crowe *et al* included in their protocols an assessment of the emotions associated with stammering. They suggested that this assessment should only be used with children over the age of 9 years in whom an emotional component has been demonstrated to be part of their stammering. They were also of the opinion that it is important that the parent is informed, because of the possibility that a parent might feel that such an assessment will heighten negative emotions about stammering. The scale consists of 40 statements, each with three possible answers ('never', 'sometimes', 'always'). Scores are totalled to give ratings on 12 different emotions – for example, shame, anxiety, denial. Ratings range from 'unnoticeable' to 'handicapping'. Crowe *et al* suggested that the assessment should be repeated during therapy, in order to monitor changes that occur.

Avoidance Behaviours

◆ *Avoidance behaviours* (Crowe *et al*, 2000) This was the subject of a further assessment proposed by Crowe's group. It comprises five sections (people, general situations, words, emotional situations, competitive and creative endeavours and 'other'). The first four sections each contain 10 statements about avoidance in the specific area, to which the response can be 'never', 'sometimes' or 'always'. The final section is left blank for the child to add any other areas of avoidance specific to him or her not already covered in the other sections. Responses from each section can be totalled and averaged to provide an overall 6-point level of avoidance score for each section and for 'overall avoidance'.

Stress

◆ Our experience shows us that some of the children who present in our clinics have experienced a great deal of change. For some, the changes have been close together (birth of a baby, starting school, moving house); for others they have been more obviously traumatic (death of a loved one, parental disharmony, burglary). Research by Yairi (2000) showed that the onset of stammering in around 50 per cent of children took place close in time to physical or emotional stress. We always ask parents about life events that could be stressful for the child. Our aim in therapy is, if possible, to try to reduce potentially stress-producing events (for example, by not introducing a new childminder as soon as a new baby is born). If this is not feasible, we would aim to help parents modify the impact such changes may have on the child

◆ *The Holmes Social Readjustment Scale for Children* (Holmes & Masuda, 1974) is one way of identifying possible stressors. It lists 43 life changes, each scoring a specific number of points. The highest score is 100 (death of a parent) and the lowest score 11 (punishment for not telling the truth). Total scores indicate levels of stress: 150 is considered average; 300+ is considered heavy stress.

Other

Crowe *et al* (2000) also outlined assessments for the following areas:

◆ Self-image
◆ Degree of handicap
◆ Perceptions of stuttering
◆ Cognitive indicators of stuttering severity
◆ Situational ratings
◆ Speech locus of control.

PARENTAL ASSESSMENTS

The battery of assessments published by Crowe *et al* (2000) contains a number of assessments for parents to complete. The authors suggested three reasons why parents should complete assessments:

1   The child is too young to complete the corresponding child assessments.

2   To identify parents whose perceptions are different from those of their children.

3   To decide if parental counselling is needed.

Attitudes and Emotions

In addition to more general assessments of the child's overt speech difficulties, reactions of family and friends, perceptions about stammering and the speaking demands the child is faced with, there are two further assessments which investigate parental attitudes and emotions about stammering. We outline these in more detail here.

◆   *Attitudes towards stuttering* (Crowe *et al*, 2000). This contains 25 statements with which parents are asked to agree or disagree. Crowe *et al* perceived this assessment as being useful as a means of initiating discussion, rather than as a pure assessment of attitudes. From our experience, we would not advise giving this to parents without allowing them an opportunity to explain their responses. Many of the answers cannot fall simply into an 'agree' or 'disagree' format. A couple of examples are 'children who stutter should not be required by teachers to speak in class' and 'it is usually best for parents to ignore their child's stuttering'. Clearly, it is possible and preferable to both agree and disagree with these statements. One of our parents who completed this assessment pointed out her dilemma in being permitted only one response to some of these questions. For example, with regard to the second example above, she agreed that parents should not continually offer advice to a child, but rather listen to the 'what' of the child's talking. However, she also saw it as unhelpful for a parent to treat stammering as a taboo subject, only to be referred to in hushed voices or out of the child's presence.

◆ *Emotional responses to stuttering* (Crowe *et al*, 2000). This assessment comprises 30 statements, each of which is rated on a 6-point scale from 0 (never) to 6 (always). As with the child assessment of the same name, scores are tallied according to specific categories, with an average rating for each. Once again, we think it is important for parents to be given the opportunity to discuss their ratings with the clinician, although we feel that the answers in this assessment are less equivocal than in the previous one.

SELF-RATING SCALES

The formal scales that we have considered so far are evaluated by the clinician. Wright & Ayre (2000) have designed a self-rating profile known as *The Wright & Ayre Stuttering Self-Rating Profile (WASSP)*. This was designed for adults who stammer, and reliability studies were carried out using this age group. However, the authors have used it clinically with people over the age of 14, and suggest that clinicians use their own judgement as to whether it is appropriate for their child patients of this age. The authors' rationale for a self-rating scale is that the client's perception of his or her overt and covert stammering and of any changes made in therapy are of prime importance. The WASSP comprises five subscales addressing the following areas, which combine overt and covert symptoms:

◆ Behaviours – for example, frequency, duration, struggle, loss of eye contact
◆ Thoughts – negative thoughts before, during and after speaking
◆ Feelings about stuttering
◆ Avoidance – as in Sheehan's (1975) five levels
◆ Disadvantage – at home, socially, educationally, at work.

Clients complete a rating sheet before a block of therapy, and the same sheet after the block. Ratings for each question on each scale are on a scale of 1 (none) to 7 (very severe). This process takes around 5 minutes. Discussion of the profile by the client and clinician is seen as paramount.

SWINDON FLUENCY PACKS

At this point we would like to mention briefly the work that has been developed by Claire McNeil and her speech and language therapy colleagues in Swindon. As described more fully in Chapter 9, this team has developed three programmes for children (Smoothies for ages 7–9 years, Blockbusters for ages 9–12 years, and Teens Challenge for ages 13–17 years) (McNeil *et al*, 2003). Each pack is accompanied by assessments for children, parents and clinicians, appropriate to the age of the children concerned. The Smoothies pack, for example, measures outcomes using three pictures of faces (sad, happy and in-between) to measure three areas – contentment with speech, enjoyment of talking and smoothness of speech. For older children, assessments are more involved, covering attitudes and behaviours to stammering, and looking at specific speaking situations. Although there are no normative data for these assessments, we have found them to measure the things which appear to be of most importance to clients, carers and clinicians, and to provide valuable pre- and post-assessment data.

CONCLUSION

In this chapter we have looked at a variety of assessments for both the overt and covert aspects of stammering in children. We leave it to clinicians to choose those most appropriate to their own clinical settings, requirements of the service, time constraints and, most importantly, the specific child concerned.

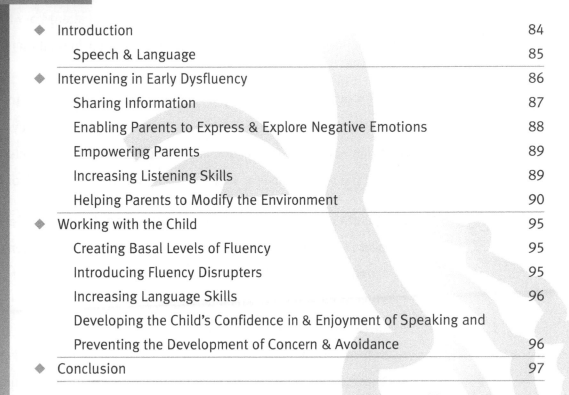

INTRODUCTION

In this chapter, we will be looking at a stage of dysfluency that usually occurs in the pre-school years. Since the first edition of *Working with Dysfluent Children* was written, there has been a great deal of research into the development of stammering (see Chapter 3) which has informed and altered our thinking. Our term 'early dysfluency' has now been defined more closely in relation to recent research.

Children in this category may or may not be more dysfluent than many of their peers, but the dysfluencies are qualitatively similar. The key to this stage of development is in our fifth dimension – the psychological aspects. So let us look at each of the five dimensions to see what we mean when we talk of early dysfluency.

1 **Quantitative.** Here we look at measurement of frequency of dysfluency, both overall and in terms of the number of iterations per repetition, and at the length of time the dysfluency has been apparent. In order for us to consider a child to be at the early dysfluency stage, we would consider the dysfluency to have been present for less than a year. Spontaneous recovery at this stage is still very likely, and more the rule than the exception. There is likely to have been some change for the better in the dysfluency over the time since onset. It may be cyclical in nature, with the most noticeable dysfluency occuring at times when the demands on the child are greater, such as when the child is tired, over-excited, ill or upset. Overall dysfluencies can vary greatly from child to child, but will be less than those of children at the borderline stage (Yairi & Lewis, 1984).

2 **Qualitative.** We refer here to the type of dysfluencies present. A child in the early dysfluency stage will predominantly demonstrate repetitions of whole words or phrases. Where SLDs do occur, they are infrequent, with fewer than two iterations per repetition (Yairi, 1981). The silent repetition between iterations will be the longest element of the repetition (Throneberg & Yairi, 1994). Clustering of dysfluencies will be infrequent (Yairi *et al*, 1993). The child in the early dysfluency category is unlikely to be more dysfluent with particular people or in certain situations.

3   **Physical.** The early dysfluent child is mostly unaware of the dysfluency and so does not display the physical characteristics associated with trying to 'do something' about it. Repetitions are thus tension-free and unhurried.

4   **Physiological.** There will at this stage be no evidence of secondary behaviours such as associated head and neck movements, loss of eye contact and so on.

5   **Psychological.** Children in the 'early dysfluency' category do not construe their speech as problematic. They may occasionally feel that a word is difficult to say, withdraw eye contact, experience or express frustration at not being able to make their point exactly when or as quickly as they may want to, change a word or even give up what they are saying. These children do not form predictions that are based on any expectation of difficulty. In other words, any construing of the dysfluency is associated purely with the moment of dysfluency.

The early dysfluency stage may be relatively short-lived, in which case the child may return to a fluency level considered to be age-appropriate.

We have chosen to call this stage 'early dysfluency' rather than 'normal non-fluency' for a number of reasons:

◆   It does not have the SLDs associated with stammering.
◆   This stage may be absent altogether (see Chapter 3 on the development of stammering). The child may start stammering at a borderline stage.
◆   Although we know so much more about the onset and development of stammering, we do not yet have all the answers. We can only say categorically that a child's dysfluency is 'normal' in retrospect – that is, when he has 'grown out' of it.

Speech & Language

As clinicians, we are aware that most stammering has its onset in the pre-school years, typically not from onset of speaking but at a time when a child's language is rapidly developing. As we have already said, 75 per cent of risk for stammering onset occurs before the age of 3 years 5 months, and the greatest risk occurs before 3 years (Yairi & Ambrose, 1992a, 1992b). There is much speculation as to the interface between language development and onset of dysfluency. Watkins & Yairi (1997, p385) suggested that the child's loss of fluency at such a time may imply 'potential interference or trade-offs in speech-language production'. Hill (1995) described the profile seen in some children whose language developed early but who started to stammer around their second birthday as being related to 'chronic linguistic overload'. Of course, a minority of children do not follow such a pattern and their dysfluency starts at or near the point of their first words. These are often the children that concern us as clinicians the most – perhaps because they seem to have had little or no experience of a prolonged period of fluency. It would, however, be hard to argue that language plays a part in the development of stammering in such children. Hill (1995) also suggested that stammering in these children may be associated with neurodevelopmental factors.

INTERVENING IN EARLY DYSFLUENCY

We approach intervention in early dysfluency from the same perspective as Hayhow & Levy (1989, p73), namely that 'work with parents should always come first'. Like Van Riper (1990), we acknowledge that we still know relatively little about stammering, but that most dysfluent children become fluent either because of maturation or because the child does not develop negative ways of dealing with the dysfluency. We therefore see our role with this group of children predominately in terms of prevention. Starkweather (1999, p233) wrote, 'We can prevent the complexity of stuttering from developing or if it has developed, we can undo it, untie the knots of frustration and struggle. And the younger the child is, the easier the knots are to untie.' In addition he stated (p243) '... we may have been barking up the wrong tree in seeing stuttering as a condition that needs to be removed, like a disease. It may be more fruitful to see it as a process that can take helpful or harmful directions. By joining the client in the recovery process, rather than trying to change him or her, it may be that we can be more effective.' We want to ensure that the child we identify in the early stammering category does not develop maladaptive ways of coping and that the dysfluencies remain as no more than 'tiny lags and disruptions in the timing of the complicated movements required for speech' (Van Riper, 1990, p317). We believe that, by helping parents to look at the dysfluency from a different perspective, we maximise the child's potential to increase his fluency. We are aware from research that 'a large proportion of young preschoolers stop stuttering within two years of onset without treatment and that such delays do not adversely affect treatment begun at the end of that period for those who do not stop' (Curlee & Yairi, 1998, p24). Rather than start direct treatment with the child at an early age, we prefer a least-first approach at this stage – assessing, observing and working with parents to promote a fluency-enhancing environment, followed by review and reassessment.

The following are some ideas we have found useful in working with parents.

Sharing Information

We agree with Manning (2001, p324) that 'parents should be informed at the outset that they have not caused this problem to occur and are not totally responsible for eliminating it. However, as a good deal of research has demonstrated, parents can be shown how to assist in altering the child's environment so stuttering behaviour is not maintained.' Parents have frequently been offered a variety of ideas from a wide range of people and are unsure of how to make sense of all the, often conflicting, advice they have been given. Being informed in a straightforward and honest way can in itself reduce much of the parents' anxiety and guilt. We would argue that we should also share our lack of knowledge, in order to work in a more effective partnership with parents.

Sharing what we know about risk factors in stammering is another helpful strategy with the parents of early dysfluent children. Letting them know what research is telling us about the amount and type of dysfluency that distinguishes this stage from borderline dysfluency can be very reassuring. Giving information about genetic factors, even if this is a significant consideration for the child, shows that we are working in a spirit of partnership and honesty. Helping parents consider how the child construes the dysfluency can also help them see the 'problem' in a different way. Examples of areas in which we would share information include:

◆ Risk factors (amount and type of early dysfluency compared with borderline stammering; genetic factors)

◆ Child's apparent construction of the dysfluency

◆ Exploration of worst-case scenarios ('what-ifs'?)

◆ Therapy options available now and at later stages

◆ Examples of children and adults who stammer but lead fulfilled and happy lives.

Enabling Parents to Express & Explore Negative Emotions

Parents can feel a wide range of negative emotions in connection with their child's dysfluency (for example, guilt, upset, sadness, embarrassment and anxiety). Some of these may not be overtly expressed. Many writers discuss the need to help parents modify the behaviours that these feelings can produce (Starkweather, 1987; Botterill *et al*, 1991). However, there seems to be less emphasis in the literature on the exploration of the attitudes themselves. We would suggest that a clinician who truly listens in an empathic, accepting and non-judgemental way enables the parent not only to express the feelings, but also to examine their validity. Negative emotions such as guilt and anxiety are not constructive, but we believe that parents can most readily be helped to change if they are given time and space to explore and understand their feelings first.

Van Riper (1973, p418) expressed his concern that so-called 'counselling' of parents by clinicians all too often consists of advice giving. This may well achieve little other than an increased feeling of guilt, fostered by a belief that it is what they have done which has been instrumental in causing the stammer. Van Riper, instead, tried 'to give parents some immediate absolution for any communicative sins of the past'. Our own approach to counselling is based on the person-centred 'core conditions' in the therapeutic relationship, namely congruence, unconditional positive regard and accurate empathic understanding (Corey, 1991). However, our practice is eclectic, and we draw techniques from a variety of psychotherapeutic models.

Starkweather & Gottwald (1990, p152) have found that group sessions for parents can provide 'emotional support as parents deal with feelings that are often paralysing'. In addition, they suggested that, when clinicians supply information in such a forum, parents gain a feeling of control which in itself can lessen some of the emotional load they carry.

Empowering Parents

Our belief is that we should work in partnership with parents. Therapy should be a collaborative venture, with each partner bringing along ideas, beliefs and feelings about the child and the problem. While these often differ, if the clinician has a fundamental respect for the parent and is prepared to listen and try to understand their construction of events, differences can be more readily explored, experiments set up and results evaluated.

Most of us who are parents have been in situations in which we have shared our concerns about our child with an empathic listener. Often, we discover our own solutions as we really hear what we are feeling, possibly for the first time. Knowing that there is someone else who understands how we are feeling and is prepared to listen but not judge us can be very reassuring. We also find that parents often experience an enormous sense of relief when they find that there is someone with whom they can share part of the burden they are carrying in their attempts to help their child. To know that they are being taken seriously, are no longer alone and that the clinician will be there when needed can in itself enable parents to let go of much of their anxiety.

Increasing Listening Skills

When parents are concerned about an aspect of their child's development, it can easily become the focus of their interaction with the child. Helping parents to alter the focus from how the child speaks onto what the child is saying can be a powerful way of changing the way they perceive the problem: not only do they cease to demonstrate their discomfort both verbally and non-verbally, but they also discover new things about their child which their hitherto constricted view was preventing. They may, for example, notice that the child has a vivid imagination, a good vocabulary or can tell a good story. As the dysfluency becomes less central to their construing of the child, they become more relaxed and less anxious about it. The child, in turn, can become less likely to construe the dysfluency as a problem.

Helping Parents to Modify the Environment

Reducing fluency disrupters

In Chapter 1 we have already discussed factors in the environment that are generally believed to disrupt a child's fluency. Helping a parent identify which of these factors may be important for their own child must be done carefully in order not to increase any feelings of guilt. There are a variety of ways in which this can be carried out, and we need to use our understanding of individual parents in choosing the most appropriate ones. Van Riper (1973) approached the task as a joint problem solver with the parents, setting observation tasks, providing information and sometimes arranging meetings with other parents who have successfully modified their own dysfluent child's speaking environment. Peters & Guitar (1991) followed a similar approach, explaining the meaning of the term 'fluency disrupters' and giving general examples. They, too, encourage parents to become good observers of their children's dysfluency and to experiment for themselves to find ways of modifying the environment. Botterill *et al* (1991, p66) advocated the use of video recordings, explaining to parents that 'the purpose of this exercise is to make some changes in the interpersonal communications that may assist the child in becoming more fluent'. Clinicians comment positively about the interaction, but also help the parents to identify one disrupter which they feel can be changed without too much difficulty. The video is then used to practise this new behaviour before it is gradually transferred into the home environment. Some parents may be helped in this process by reading material. There are some excellent pamphlets and books in publication which we can recommend or lend to parents (available from the British Stammering Association). We would suggest, however, that these are used as an adjunct. They should not be handed out without prior discussion as to how they may be used, or without an opportunity to explore parents' reactions once they have been read.

Increasing situations that enhance fluency

Most young children, however severe their dysfluency, have times at which they are almost always fluent. These occasions may vary between children, but we have found the following to be quite common:

◆ Playing alone with toys

◆ Singing/saying nursery rhymes

◆ Talking to pets

◆ Using simple speech

◆ Speaking in unison

◆ Talking when there is plenty of time

◆ Playing in a one-to-one situation with a parent

◆ Being in a non-competitive or quiet speaking environment without distractions.

Using rating scales (such as those in the Lidcombe Programme or as referred to in Chapter 4) can help parents to identify times at which their child tends to be more dysfluent. The parents can be asked to focus on listening to the child's dysfluency during a specific activity for about 10–15 minutes per day (taking a different daily activity wherever possible) and to bring these ratings to the clinic to explore them with the clinician to see if any patterns can be noted. These can then be the basis for experimentation. Some children are more dysfluent when they are tired. If this is so, then altering bedtimes or introducing a nap may help. For others, over-excitement may be linked with the dysfluency. Experiments in such cases could involve not telling the child as soon about a planned activity, or spreading out fun things rather than having several such occurrences in close succession.

Parents, understandably, often say that they feel a need to 'do' something about the child's speech, hence the reason that they often offer advice to 'slow down', 'take a deep breath', and so on, even when they acknowledge that often this may only serve to annoy and frustrate the child. We have found that this frequently occurs when one of the child's parents has or has had a stammer and desperately wants to stop their child undergoing a similar experience. We recall a parent with a stammer who had, many years previously, attended one of our prolonged speech courses. His solution for his three-year-old son was to teach him the same technique. Helping a parent to modify the child's speaking environment fulfils a much needed role for a parent to be proactive and help the child in a more constructive way.

In much the same way in which parents are asked to identify fluency disrupters, they can be asked to try to discover if there are situations in which their child is more likely to be fluent. They may then be able to create these situations more frequently. In addition, Peters & Guitar (1991) suggested that parents can respond to the cyclical nature of the child's stammering. When the child's speech is more fluent, the child can be encouraged to talk more. At more dysfluent times, quieter, fluency-enhancing activities may be increased.

Using the demands & capacities model

We find this a most useful model to discuss with parents. (Refer to Chapter 2 for a detailed explanation of the model, and the diagram we use to explain it to parents.) Used carefully and appropriately, it helps in our aim of reducing guilt and increasing empowerment. Parents can see that there are a number of factors involved in dysfluency and a variety of ways in which the child can be helped.

We spend one or more sessions with parents, looking at each section of the model and its relevance to their individual child. We describe each section in non-technical language and ask the parents to tell us about their perceptions of its relevance to their child. As an example, let us take the section on psychological factors. We ask about the child's personality: How would each parent describe the child? Who is the child most like? What sort of personality is developing? Is the child active or passive? Does he lead or follow? How does he cope with change? How do the parents introduce changes?

Together, we set up experiments to see what, if anything, seems to make a difference. If, for example, we discover that the child finds change difficult, we might suggest that the family try to explain new things in more detail. We might tell them the story of a child we worked with who was moving house and became very upset. His parents eventually found out why – he had thought that moving house meant leaving behind, not only the house, but his precious possessions too. We may suggest that changes are spaced out, or not 'hyped up' for weeks in advance. Each child and each family is different, and any experiments have to be meaningful, relevant and 'do-able'. J's mother, for example, felt that the most enjoyable part of being a parent was the excitement and build-up to forthcoming events. She needed to have something to look forward to, and would tell J about it weeks before. J's father, a much more easy-going and laid-back individual, found this quite difficult and there was a feeling that J did too. J's mother could not, nor did she want to, change her behaviour – for her, it would have taken away a lot of the joy of parenting. However, she was able to delay telling J *quite* as soon and to give J some idea of how long the wait would be by introducing the concept of the number of 'sleeps' before the big event.

Gottwald (1999, p183) proposed a way forward. She suggested looking at the child's fluency environment from a systems perspective, and working holistically with the family, not looking at 'individual or static segments such as parent speech rate or family turn-taking behavior, but at the relationship of these segments and the interaction of these segments with one another'. In addition, she pointed out that different families are differently able to put changes in their interaction patterns into practice. She suggested that clinicians should balance therapy between capacities and demands according to the parents' belief in the benefits of environmental changes and their ability to translate ideas into behaviours. We are very aware of this in our therapy. One family was keen to look at ways in which they might modify their interactions and, indeed, had started to do so instinctively before even coming for therapy. Another family coping with a myriad of demands could not take on changes, and preferred the clinician to take all responsibility for enhancement of fluency. In this family, we worked directly with the child in school, using a support worker.

Gottwald (p179) neatly summed up possible environmental influences as follows:

◆ Parent speech behaviours
◆ Rate of fluent speech
◆ Pace of conversation
◆ Kind and number of questions
◆ Length and complexity of sentences.

Family interaction patterns:

◆ Turn-taking
◆ Quality time for talking
◆ Topic initiations and changes
◆ Request for verbal performance.

Family reactions to stuttering:

◆ Negative comments
◆ Instructions to speak otherwise
◆ Negative feelings expressed implicitly.

Family lifestyle characteristics:

◆ Structured versus unstructured
◆ High versus low expectations
◆ Stable versus unstable
◆ Clear versus confusing discipline.

We are also honest about the contradictory research findings, but tell parents about strategies that we believe, from our clinical experience, are worth 'having a go' at. If, for example, we feel that a parent's speech may be too fast for the child, we suggest experimenting with slowing their own speech rate. We acknowledge that this is a very difficult task, especially for a habitually fast speaker. We need to help the parent with suggestions as to ways of actually slowing down:

◆ Use pauses
◆ Do not speak straight away in response to a question or enquiry from the child
◆ Take more time to breathe
◆ Use thinking time during an utterance
◆ Use slow articulatory contacts.

Some parents find some of these methods easier than others. These experiments will enable them to find a method that is most helpful to them personally.

If parents find it hard to tolerate interruptions, we discuss how hard it is for a child to 'hold on' to their thoughts and how parents can allow the child to interrupt them more.

WORKING WITH THE CHILD

As we have already stated, we rarely work directly with the child who we consider to be in an early dysfluency stage, preferring to empower the parents to be the prime force for change. However, we would consider this step if work on modification of the environment has been tried and failed (for whatever reason) or if parents could not/would not cooperate.

In working with the young child who is unaware of his dysfluency, we are essentially undertaking a preventative role. We aim to ensure that he does not develop a feeling that his speech is unacceptable in some way. We would also hope to increase his capacity for fluent speech. Some of the following ideas may be useful for working with the child at this stage:

Creating Basal Levels of Fluency

In creating basal levels of fluency, we are aiming to give the child as much experience of fluency as possible. We have outlined above some of the most likely situations in which a child may be fluent and find talking pleasurable. By providing these in the clinic, we are not only giving the child an enjoyable speaking experience, but we are also modelling appropriate interventions for the parents (by speaking slowly and simply, asking few questions, not interrupting, and so on).

Introducing Fluency Disrupters

Once we have established basal levels of fluency, we start very gradually to introduce possible fluency disrupters, to ascertain whether they have any effect on the child's fluency. We could, for example, speak more quickly or ask more questions. As we do so, we need to observe the child's reaction and the effect on fluency, in order to judge their significance for a particular child. When dysfluency occurs, we return to basal levels. Hayhow & Levy (1989) suggested the following ways of increasing demands made on the child:

◆ Increasing the number of people present
◆ Introducing background noise
◆ Interruptions and surprises
◆ Use of contradictions
◆ Time pressure
◆ Increasing emotional significance of material
◆ Competition
◆ Changing location.

These must be carefully structured, in order both to help us to ascertain the effect they have on fluency and to increase the child's tolerance of such disrupters.

Increasing Language Skills

There has, over the years, been much debate as to whether language skills should be worked on if the child is also dysfluent. There has been a widespread fear that so doing will increase the severity of the dysfluency. We would argue that, if poor language skills are reducing a child's capacity for fluent speech, then working on them might serve to increase this capacity. Obviously, the child's fluency while such work is being undertaken should be closely monitored to ascertain if there is indeed any consequent effect on dysfluency. Should this occur, the level at which the intervention is taking place may need to be reviewed. However, to ignore the language difficulties seems to us to limit the child's potential for developing effective communication.

Developing the Child's Confidence in & Enjoyment of Speaking and Preventing the Development of Concern and Avoidance

For most young children, speaking is fun. If we feel that it is helpful to work with a young child, we want to ensure that this enjoyment continues. Consequently, activities must reinforce positive experiences when talking. By showing that we find communicating with the child enjoyable, we can reinforce the child's self-esteem. By attending to content, and responding to the *what* and not the *how* of talking, we can help the child to see his contribution as valuable. If he is receiving other messages in his home environment, then our intervention may help to contradict some of the negative input he is receiving.

CONCLUSION

It is our belief that we should always work with parents of a child whom we assess to be in the early stammering category. On occasions, we may also decide to work with the child. When the child is not aware of any difficulties in speaking, the intervention should be supportive, fluency enhancing and aim to prevent the development of secondary symptoms. We would rarely advocate teaching of specific fluency techniques, either directly or indirectly, at this early stage.

Chapter 6: Borderline Stammering

DEFINING THE CATEGORY

As we see it, the key to our use of the term 'borderline stammerer' is children's construing of their non-fluent experiences, and not necessarily a measurable change in the quantifiable and qualitative dimensions that Yairi and his colleagues have described (see Chapter 3). There may, however, be changes in the physical presentation of the dysfluency and the temporal characteristics that Yairi and his group outline in the physical and physiological dimensions. It is our belief that these are responses to an underlying change in children's psychological dimensions – their emotional responses to the dysfluencies of which they are increasingly aware.

So what might a child with a borderline stammer look like? Let us create a picture by applying Yairi's dimensions and our own fifth dimension:

1 **Quantitative – the measurement of frequency and duration of dysfluency, and number of iterations in repetitions**

    Children at this stage are likely to have moved out of the period when we would expect spontaneous recovery, so are likely to be at least 18 months to 2 years post onset. The pattern of the frequency of the dysfluency has probably shown little change over a number of months, perhaps even since onset, and in some cases may be worsening (that is, the percentage of dysfluent syllables has increased).

2 **Qualitative – different types of dysfluency (SLDs as opposed to other dysfluencies), clustering of dysfluencies**

    Qualitatively, we often see a pattern similar to the previous dimension, with the number of SLDs remaining significantly high (in relation to the other types of dysfluencies), or increasing in certain situations or for certain periods of time.

    In addition, there can be a subtle shift in the types of dysfluencies experienced. For example, there may be a move from repetitions to prolongations and/or blocks which precipitate problems initiating speech or give rise to difficulties in maintaining speech flow. There may be attempts to shorten the duration of the non-fluency by decreasing the length of the repetitions and/or increasing the tempo of the iterations (see physical dimension, below).

3 Physical – temporal characteristics, rate of repetitions

If children have, as we assert, become more aware and concerned by their dysfluencies, it is likely that there will be changes in this physical dimension. We suggest that this will be linked to the presence of tension and struggle. Symptoms that indicate the presence of tension include prolonged vowels with or without a rise in vocal pitch, increased loudness associated with non-fluencies, and general struggle behaviour.

As we have indicated before, the increased awareness accompanied by a decrease in children's tolerance of dysfluency may also lead to the shortening of the dysfluencies by increasing the rate of the iterations.

4 Physiological – associated behaviours (head and neck movements), tension

In this dimension, we may see changes associated with struggle and tension. Yairi and his colleagues have discussed the frequency of head and neck movements that are particularly associated with the onset of stammering in some children. Unlike at onset, at this stage movements are not integral to stammering, but rather 'added on' by children themselves. These behaviours can be seen as children's attempts to gain more control by using other body parts which they know they can control. Thus we can see in the borderline stage the development of such secondary behaviours as loss of eye contact and foot and/or hand tapping.

5 Psychological

At this stage, children are becoming or have become aware of their dysfluencies, both within the moment and outside the event. As a result, they start to be aware of the negative implications of their stammer in terms of their speech and, more significantly, for themselves as individuals interacting with others.

What we will see that reflects this awareness and the associated negativity is the development of avoidance and/or escape behaviours (for example, use of starters, word substitution, avoiding speaking and speaking situations). There can also be some fear of stammering, which may be fleeting, or attached to specific situations or people.

In line with fluctuation in speech, we might also learn of changes in children's general pattern of behaviour. The family or school may report examples of frustration or aggression on the one hand or withdrawal or periods of isolation on the other. These can be directly associated with the non-fluencies or observed over longer periods without the cause being readily identifiable. There may also be changes in relationships at this point. Some friendships become strained or difficult and some children lose friends without the reason apparently being associated with communication difficulties.

We may also see significant changes in the way children construe themselves. Difficulties in fluency can be transferred as children begin to construe that they have difficulties in other areas and are unable to do activities they previously carried out without a moment's thought. At this stage we should be aware that children have an increased sense of self and a heightened sensitivity. This may make them acutely aware of any perceived shortcomings or criticisms.

BORDERLINE STAMMERING AT PRIMARY SCHOOL AGE

Unlike some theorists and practitioners, we are reluctant to assign chronological age norms to this developmental stage. In our clinical work, we have met children as young as two and a half years who appear to be at this stage, and some who present in this way from the onset of dysfluencies. In contrast, there are other children who have remained within this phase until adolescence. However, we are aware of developments in construing around the age of 6–8 years, with individuals appearing to reconstrue themselves and their non-fluencies. This may not be typical, but certainly several clients we have met have experienced a change at this stage.

We propose to look at borderline stammering, taking this age group as an example, and demonstrate how we might examine children's view of themselves and their environment and relate those observations to the changes they are demonstrating and reporting in their speech.

FACTORS TO CONSIDER IN THE BORDERLINE STAMMERER

Children's reconstruction of speech does not happen in isolation, and we must take a holistic view of the child and consider what factors may be triggering change within that child. In our discussions with children and their families, we attempt to identify what might be different in their particular situation and possibly have precipitated this development. Depending on the age of the child, different factors may be significant. The following are suggestions of areas to consider for primary school children.

Self

As always, our starting point is the child in front of us in clinic. In order to be effective and design a management plan which will be appropriate for him, we need to know what he thinks about the problem and about himself as a person. It is interesting to look at how balanced a view he has of himself; whether for example, his speech difficulty is offset by being in the school football team, with the associated 'street credibility' that comes with it. We should also be prepared for the concrete nature of construing. This has come home to us in relation to our own children. When asked to describe himself, *S* at six and a half, did not say 'talks a lot', 'energetic' or other words which, as his parent, we would have considered appropriate. Rather, he said 'I've got brown hair. I'm quite thin and I wear my socks rolled down.' We must expect the children's perceptions or lack of perceptions about themselves and their speech also to be very concrete. We were discussing 'getting stuck' with *K*, an eight-year-old non-fluent girl and asked, 'Do you ever get stuck on your words, *K*?'. 'Oh, yes!' she said. Attempting to examine her construing further, we continued, 'What do you do when that happens?'. 'I just go and ask my Mum what the word says,' came the reply. Obviously, she related getting stuck to reading, and did not appear to construe her speech as a difficulty. Thus if the child does not construe his speech as a problem, perhaps it is not one.

Language

We know that, at this age, children's language skills are well developed. We could say that children produce language almost at an automatic level; for example, one rarely hears children searching for words or struggling with a structure to convey their intent at this stage unless they have a specific word-finding or syntactical problem. This is one area that we should examine, therefore, to see if their capacities are age-appropriate.

Demands are being made on children in terms of the expectations of those around them – expectations which may be based on performance levels of children of a similar age, such as national norms. It may be that borderline-stammering children do not have age-appropriate language levels and struggle to cope, or it could be the children themselves who are setting unrealistically high language targets.

One young girl, A, began to have difficulties with her speech when she started attending a private school. Having previously coped reasonably well, she found herself competing with very articulate and assertive girls. A's language skills, observed to be age-appropriate, were no longer adequate in this group, and she struggled both socially and with her fluency.

We also know that, at primary school age, specific demands are made on children's speech at school (for example, reading out loud in front of at least one adult and perhaps a group of peers; answering questions in class). Registration may be stressful. Saying your name or the teacher's name in a specific format ('Yes, Miss X'), at the precise moment it is requested and in a way in which it can be heard and understood, is a situation which many of our adult clients recall with horror. The appearance of dysfluencies at that very moment may be perceived as the focus of everyone's attention.

The Peer Group

It is at this age that the peer group begins to be influential. Indeed, Turner & Helms (1991, p289) stated, 'Learning how to deal with their peers is itself one of the greatest challenges confronting children between their sixth and twelfth years.' Not only are children mixing with a variety of others at school, but in many instances nowadays children are involved in several out-of-school groups. They may attend swimming lessons, dancing classes, or join social and uniformed organisations. This increases the number of situations in which they have contact with their peers.

As with the other factors, there is no single issue relating to a child's peer group that will move him along the route to confirmed stammering. However, there are a number of points to consider:

- *Establishing relationships.* Among primary school children, the formation of relationships is important. At this time we see the sexes split into separate groups, 'best' friends are established and, a little later, leader and follower roles emerge. If our clients are unable to enter into this process, for whatever reason, we may see speech become more dysfluent. One of our clients, *A*, was delayed in terms of her social and emotional development. She was finding it hard to make friends and, as a result, was isolated from the peer group of which she wanted so much to be a part. She did not have any strategies to cope with or change the situation, other than attention-seeking behaviours, which were inappropriate and only succeeded in isolating her further. We gave her mother some ideas for role playing to help *A* deal more effectively with these social situations: for example, having a friend round for tea and playing games the friend chose, taking a toy into school to show her peers, talking to two or three children about something she watched on television or at the cinema. Thus, *A* was able to develop strategies that were socially acceptable and allowed some integration with her peer group.

- *Dynamics.* It is important to remember that boys and girls tend to have different kinds of friendships. Boys often choose friends around activities such as football, and are less likely to be dependent on one best friend. Girls, on the other hand, form more emotional relationships in which best friends can matter more and upsets in relationships can be devastating. The peer group often undergoes a change of dynamics at this stage. We hear of groups of girls falling in and out of friendships. However, it is not only girls who have difficulties. One boy, *B*, found himself in the middle of a group of boys among whom two or three were exercising control over the others. *B* found this very difficult to manage and his speech deteriorated. He was finally able to discuss this with his parents and teacher, and strategies were put in place to reduce the intimidation that he and others had experienced. Only later did he seek help for his speech. When asked why, he said he thought he needed to 'sort out the first problem before sorting out speech'.

He had obviously made the connection between the group difficulties and his speech. He was eight years old.

◆ *Group wisdom.* With this peer group contact, there comes the growing realisation that Mum, Dad and/or teacher are not the fount of all knowledge, and peers have a contribution to make. Children begin at this stage to report the opinions of friends as fact: 'Alan says you are allowed to take toys to school.' Alongside this they may also report others' beliefs, attitudes or behaviours towards themselves: 'Sam says I'm silly', or 'Thomas wouldn't play with me at break time.' We acknowledge the need for children to take account of the views of others.

◆ *Reconstruing self.* Group wisdom can become the main agent for reconstruing of self. On one hand the peer group can be powerful and work positively, giving children knowledge and awareness of what is socially acceptable and enabling them to develop the skill of self-evaluation. Alternatively, it can be destructive if children's performances are perceived as unacceptable or inferior when compared with others they view as important models.

◆ *Reconstruction of dysfluencies.* In terms of non-fluencies it is our experience that the peer group has often been the precipitating factor for several clients' reconstruction. A casual remark like 'Why do you talk funny?', or more malicious teasing or imitating children's speech can play a large part in drawing stammering to children's attention. Because of the importance of the peer group at this stage, these remarks may be crucial in beginning the reconstruction of dysfluencies into stammering. It is worthwhile considering the group's attitude towards fluency, and their actual levels of fluent or non-fluent speech. Some writers report less tolerance towards dysfluency in highly fluent groups. In our experience, there is much variability: some groups with less fluent members can focus on dysfluent children as scapegoats and perhaps use them as a target for some of their own frustrations, whereas others are very tolerant and understanding. It is important to gain information on the group as a whole; individual group members may report attitudes that differ from the group when interviewed individually, but in the group situation will conform to the group norm.

◆ *Group's attitude to and use of speech and language.* If we accept that the peer group has an important part to play in children's level of fluency, then the group's use of speech and language, their level of fluency and their attitudes towards communication must be considered. We should try to obtain information on the level of language used by the group and compare it with that of our client to see if they are interacting and possibly competing in a group with a level comparable to their own. If the group's use of syntax and vocabulary is above our client's then, as encountered in the family, the child may struggle both to understand and to express himself. This could tip the child's language balance in favour of non-fluency.

Dysfluent children may also feel pressure resulting from the speed of exchange within the group. Group interactions are often characterised by quick repartee, interruptions and talking before a person's turn has been completed. If children have problems taking turns or initiating speech generally, they may be tense and/or anxious in groups and feel 'swamped' in any interaction.

The Environment

Family and home

In previous chapters we have discussed important factors in the speech and general behaviour of the family. One area that is worthy of further comment in terms of primary school children is that of frequent change. Change is always difficult, but for children who are on the brink of stammering such difficulties need even more careful handling. We have known some families for whom family life is just one long event, where there is always something for children to get excited about, be it the visit of a friend or relative or an outing to some attraction or place of interest. Under normal circumstances such a family life could be fun and rich, but for borderline stammering children it is worth considering whether this sustained level of excitement is beyond their capacity. It may be that the levels of tension these activities produce contribute to the dysfluency the child experiences and that, if these were reduced, then correspondingly their fluency may increase. Another approach to this problem could be to help children themselves cope better with change and excitement. The use of some relaxation time or discussion with the family about the forthcoming events, and looking at ways of preparing children for the events which are planned, may improve children's abilities to cope with family life.

A final issue, again mentioned previously, is the focus of the problem. We must consider whose problem the dysfluencies actually are. If the child says they do not worry him, then perhaps the child's speech serves to take the family's attention off another problem area. It might be part of our therapeutic role to help the family identify this possibility and then deal with it in a constructive way.

School and teachers

As children progress through school they are faced with numerous cognitive, social and emotional challenges. With each new class, they have to adapt to an altered routine, conform to a different regime and learn to relate to a new leader at the front of the class. This obviously places great demands on their growing capacities in a number of key areas, and if they feel overwhelmed by the situation it is likely that fluency will suffer. In particular, the classroom teacher exerts a strong influence on children's behaviour and attitudes in all sorts of ways. It is an accepted fact that 'teacher behaviour affects pupil performance' (Turner & Helms, 1991). One of the factors that we as clinicians must consider, therefore, is the way in which that behaviour may affect the move from early dysfluent speech to stammering speech.

There are a number of key areas relevant to schools and teachers; these are fully developed in later chapters.

THE INTERVENTION

The final group of factors to consider is related to the nature of the intervention. Given the age group we are considering, we should be aware that this may be the parents' first contact with speech and language therapy. Often, they have left the child's non-fluency untreated on the advice of a medical practitioner and/or believing that the child would grow out of it. Now they come to clinic with uncertainty that this approach has been correct; perhaps it will not go away? Any intervention we are involved in must be better than this 'leave it alone' policy. It should be 'the difference that makes the difference'.

It is not easy to define therapy and predict outcomes in the best of clinical circumstances, but with borderline stammering it is especially difficult. Nevertheless, we must be clear about the aims and objectives of therapy. Will therapy improve the child's level of control over and attitude to his speech? Or will it perhaps worsen the situation by focusing attention on speech, and reinforcing parents' views and those of teachers that there is a problem to be managed and ultimately controlled? In relation to the child, will he be helped by speech and language therapy, or will it only change his construing of himself to someone with a speech problem, someone who needs help to change?

THERAPY OPTIONS

In considering some therapy options, we embrace the 'least first' philosophy; that is, tailoring any intervention to fit the child and his situation and only doing the minimal amount necessary to facilitate change. The following therapeutic choices are only a selection from which clinicians might choose. They are also not mutually exclusive, and will be used in addition to work on identification and management of demands and capacities.

Total Communication

The focus for therapy might be all the features of 'good talking'. The clinician could, therefore, outline the process of communication with discussion of both verbal and non-verbal behaviour. Together, the client and clinician might look at a different area of communication each week – facial expression, eye contact, use of gesture, articulation of speech, speech rate, and so on. In this approach, non-fluency or stammering is not of direct concern.

Here are some ideas therapists might use for different aspects of communication.

Eye contact

1 **Blindfold conversation**. Two participants have a conversation, first with both blindfolded and then with only one having a blindfold. A third person or therapist acts as an observer. At the end of the conversations, participants and observer discuss the differences in the conversations and changes in behaviour that may have occurred in the absence of eye contact.

2 **Wink murder**. Participants sit in a circle. One participant has secretly been nominated the 'murderer'. He 'murders' other group members by winking at them. They can 'die' in amusing and dramatic ways, but must have their eyes shut for the duration of the game following their death. Another participant acts as the 'detective', and must try to identify the murderer before he wipes out the whole group. This game helps children to keep eye contact within a group setting, and they are rewarded for their efforts.

3 **Contact on the first word**. Two participants engage in a question-and-answer activity. At the beginning of each utterance/response, they have to make eye contact while saying the first word.

4 **Notice colour**. Participants have to have 10 conversations with different people. The aim is to notice the eye colour of each of the other people and feed back this information to the therapist.

Facial expression

1 **'In the manner of'**. Each person is given a number of sentences to say/read aloud. Each sentence has to be said conveying a different emotion or feeling, such as anger, fear or excitement. Observers may be asked to guess what emotion is being conveyed. Groups may discuss the behaviours which enabled the emotion to be communicated successfully. The activity is then repeated with each participant using facial expression to convey an emotion, this time without saying the sentence.

Here are some sentences which may be used:

(a) Children don't get enough pocket money from their parents these days

(b) The alien spacecraft was just metres away from Alastair's front door

(c) She could hardly believe her eyes when she opened the door to her room

(d) Out of the darkness, the figure gradually took a sinister shape

(e) The team managed a shot in the last minute of extra time, to win the game.

2 **Use cards with individuals or groups showing different emotions**. These cards, which are available commercially, can be used to stimulate discussion on when and where children have experienced similar emotions. They can also be used to help children understand the expressions required to convey particular emotions and cue them in to use them in communication games.

3 **Look at soaps/sitcoms with the sound turned off**. Using taped examples from a television series, participants are asked to look at particular interactions and consider what is being expressed and how the characters are using facial expression to achieve this.

4 **Give emotion and create still life/tableau**. Participants are given a particular emotion, such as fear or care, and asked to illustrate this using a tableau. Appropriate facial expressions and body postures are encouraged. Observers from other groups may be asked to guess what is being illustrated.

Use of gesture

1 **Have a conversation using gestures only**. Two participants may choose to wear blank masks, but the main aim of the task is to have a conversation using only gestures. Individuals have to:

(a) Find out the time

(b) Find the way out

(c) Ask the other their name

(d) Ask where the nearest café is

(e) Ask if they can take the other person's photograph.

2 **Role-play exaggerated use of gesture**. Participants use exaggerated gestures in the following scenarios:

(a) The doctor's/dentist's waiting room with a long queue

(b) A café serving poor food

(c) A teacher and an unruly classroom

(d) A family entertaining some visitors from another country

(e) Some children working out how to play a game.

3 **Acting as another person's hands and arms**. One participant in a pair stands behind their partner and threads their arms through so they look and behave as the other person's arms. (The front person in the pair must put their arms behind the first person's back if the full effect is to be achieved.) The person in the front then recounts a story or event and the 'arms' must act in the context of the story, with appropriate gestures in time with the speaker's tale and emphasis. Examples of stories are as follows:

(a) Getting up late

(b) Going on holiday

(c) Putting on make-up

(d) Going swimming

(e) A family celebration.

Body language

1 **Different levels**. Participants role-play different situations, which usually involve characters adopting different positions in relation to the other(s). In this activity, participants should experiment with being in the contrary position as well as adopting the usual positions. Examples of scenarios include:

(a) Naughty child interviewed by headmaster

(b) Small child trying to get their busy mother's attention

(c) Buying an item when the shop assistant is behind a counter

(d) Giving a talk to a small group of people

(e) A person in hospital receiving visitors.

(It is interesting to notice how the use of language changes when different positions are taken. Individuals have difficulty adopting the usual roles in these situations.)

2 **Back to back**. In pairs, participants position themselves back-to-back and have a conversation without being able to see the other person's body

language (or facial expression). Therapists may need to cue children into what messages they are NOT getting. Examples of topics to be discussed:

(a) The day my pet died

(b) If I ruled the world

(c) What it is like having parents like mine

(d) The worst holiday I have had

(e) What it is like having to go to my school.

3 **Sit, stand, bend**. In groups of three, participants have to depict a scene using three positions, one sitting, one standing and one in between, or another position. The therapist or other groups of children can be invited to discuss the appropriateness of the positions adopted in relation to the roles as set out in the tableau.

4 **Frozen moments**. In groups of three or four, participants act out particular scenes. At an appropriate moment the therapist or member from another group shouts 'freeze'. The group has to hold their body positions at that moment and then on the command 'thaw', they start another scene from the positions in which they were frozen. A further option is that another group adopts the 'frozen' positions and starts their scene from that point. Examples of starting improvisations:

(a) Practising for the school play

(b) A family getting ready for Gran coming to stay

(c) Bonfire night in the garden

(d) It's your birthday!

(e) Who left the bath tap running?

Articulation of speech

1 **Hard attack**. After modelling by the clinician, children are asked to consider when hard attack might be used under normal circumstances – what type of words, what type of situations, with what people, to depict what feelings (for example, army commands, in emergency situations, where people are in danger, when someone is angry)?

2   **Soft attack**. After modelling by the clinician, children are asked to consider when soft attack might be used – what type of words, situations, with whom, to depict what feelings (for example, getting a baby to sleep, when stroking an animal, reading a bedtime story, in a library, when saying you love someone)?

3   **Contrasts**. After modelling by the clinician, children are asked to practise hard and soft attack at word level. Word-level activities include many guessing games used with children, such as 'I spy', or 'What am I thinking?'. In modelling, examples of words are as follows:

Hard attack	Soft attack
Go	Sleepy
Stop	Quiet
No	Whisper
Now	There
Don't	Good

4   **Sentences**. The contrast exercise above (No 3) is repeated, this time using sentences provided. Examples of appropriate sentences are as follows:

Hard attack	Soft attack
Ready, steady, go	You are such a sleepy boy
Stop right there	It's time to be quiet now
No you cannot go out in the rain	Can you whisper your answer?
You must go now	There, there
Don't do that	That's a good picture

Turn taking

1   **Dessin dicté**. In this modification of a well-used activity, a pair of children are seated either side of a divider. One child has a simple line drawing in front of them – for example, a box, a glass, a fork. The divider prevents the second child from seeing the drawing. The first child has to describe the drawing to enable the second to draw his own version. We usually do this activity twice with each pair: once when the second child is not allowed to speak, and again when he is allowed to ask clarification questions. It is during this repetition of

the task that turn-taking becomes an issue: the children have to work out when to speak, and when to be silent, to allow the drawing to be carried out.

2   **Interruptions**. Before children can manage interruptions of others and even use interruptions themselves, there needs to be a discussion about when and why interruptions occur. For example, interruptions can function constructively in a conversation to signal an emergency or some event that requires attention, and allows turn taking when one person is dominating the conversation and so on. Children can then be encouraged to look at ways in which people take others' turns. Examples include:

(a) Hand gestures

(b) Use of positive eye contact

(c) Change of body posture

(d) Appropriate vocalisation.

It is then useful for children to experiment, both using these techniques, and maintaining their turn when the techniques are used 'against' them. It is helpful to role-play these in pairs and in small group situations where possible.

Starting off conversations

Many children whom we see have difficulty in this area. Very often they are not experienced in taking responsibility for initiating communication, and do not know where to start. The clinician's role is to hand the responsibility over to the child and to resist helping them out too quickly when/if they falter. Very often, being placed in the situation can help children work out their own ways. One fun way of doing this is, in pairs or in small groups, to start off every utterance with a different letter of the alphabet in sequential order:'Are you going on holiday?' 'But I think you know I am;' 'Can you believe it's only 10 days till we break up?' 'Do you think it will go quickly?'

Maintaining conversations

In addition to the activity described in starting off conversations, which can also be used here, there are a couple of other activities which can be fun to do in pairs or with a clinician:

1   Have a conversation with no questions

2   Hold a conversation with only questions.

Ending conversations

As with many of these activities, children need some degree of preparation. In this case we encourage them to make a list of the different ways they can end a conversation. These will include a combination of gesture and appropriate language. Children like to collect examples from the television, and it often gives them a valid excuse to watch 'soaps'! They can then experiment with using different ways of ending conversations, perhaps focusing on those that they would not normally use themselves.

Following on from this, children can role-play holding conversation(s) with others, but prevent them from leaving by ending the conversation in lots of different ways, for example, 'well, see you next week then', 'love to your mother', 'take care won't you?', 'drive safely' and so on.

Volume

As with rate control, we encourage children to look at volume as something that they can change according to the situation, the content of their utterance and the emotion/intent they wish to convey. We may have them carry out an observation activity before their own experimentation, to see when people they meet speak quietly and when they speak loudly. The following activities are tasks which help children to practise different levels in different contexts:

1   Practise along a long corridor, throwing voice to a person standing increasing distances away, or at home with Mum in one room and the child in another or upstairs.

2   Practise saying quietly things that you would normally shout, such as, 'You've got to get out of here!'; 'Don't do that, you'll hurt yourself.'

3   Practise saying loudly things that you would normally whisper, such as, 'Is she asleep?', or (in a Maths lessons), 'Pass this note to Alastair.'

Pitch & intonation

Following a discussion with children about the use of pitch to denote intent and/or emotion, they can be encouraged to try various different pitches and intonation patterns out themselves. For example:

1   They can change the meaning (eg, a question to a statement) of the following examples:
    (a) He passed the test
    (b) She has brown eyes
    (c) Her mother is not feeling well
    (d) The team is playing away on Saturday
    (e) You have not seen your Gran since she was ill.

2   How to make something boring sound interesting:
    (a) It took such a long time
    (b) He had to do the same thing over and over
    (c) The teacher's voice droned on and on, as his eyes got heavier and heavier
    (d) She had to stay still for nearly an hour until the work was done
    (e) The clock ticked, the cat yawned, Granddad fell asleep, but the children knew there were still presents to open.

3   Using different intonation patterns, describe these mundane activities and make them interesting to someone from Mars:
    (a) Buttering bread
    (b) Bouncing a ball
    (c) Making your bed
    (d) Sweeping the floor
    (e) Washing your face
    (f) Brushing your teeth.

4   The effect of putting stress on different words in a sentence and how it can change meaning.
    (a) Leeds football team are relegated again
    (b) Probably the best food in the house
    (c) He couldn't look at her

(d) There are so many different songs

(e) She plays her instrument every day.

Openness

The second area of therapy to consider in the least-first approach is openness. Here, therapy would focus both on general communication (as in the first example) and also on the non-fluent speech behaviours. Therapy sessions may develop specific communication skills as before, but with work carried out to encourage openness about non-fluencies: avoidance reduction, intervention to reduce struggle. The clinician may help children reconstrue themselves as 'OK' people, irrespective of the levels of non-fluencies they are experiencing.

The following are some specific ideas that a clinician might use:

Openness

1 Draw a picture of your stammer

2 Talk to your best friend about famous people who stammer

3 Teach your best friend how to stammer like you

4 Write a story about a hero who stammers

5 Talk to your teacher about what happens when you get stuck in class sometimes

6 Stammer on purpose with a family member

7 Tell someone you are going for speech and language therapy.

Avoidance reduction

1 Have a general discussion with the child about how we stop doing things, for example, reducing the amount of cola you drink, cutting down on chocolate. There are often some ideas the child already has that can be put to good use.

2   Write a hierarchy of difficult situations and devise a plan for tackling them in a 'small steps' way.

3   The child writes down difficult words and practises one a day while having tea with their parent or carer.

4   If the child has difficulty saying the teacher's name, he calls his parent/carer by the teacher's name for a specified period during the day.

5   The child writes a diary of things he did which he did not avoid (could be words, situations, talking and so on). This is then shown to the parent/carer and therapist for praise/reward.

Reducing struggle

1   Videotape a conversation and play it back, looking for signs of struggle. The child decides which ones to target to reduce. The clinician assigns a specific situation in which the child can experiment with reducing this particular behaviour (ideally with an adult to monitor his efforts. The clinician can assist this process by providing an appropriate observation or checklist for the parent to use).

2   The clinician models the child's struggle behaviour in a conversation, and the child observes the clinician and indicates when he notices it happening. Roles are reversed, and the clinician monitors the child. Finally, both child and clinician engage in a conversation or game and monitor each other while trying to reduce their own struggle behaviour. This can also be done with small groups of children.

3   A variant of the above activity can be played when a physical behaviour is being worked on. The monitor uses small post-it notes or stickers, which are applied to the person/child when examples of the behaviour are noticed. The winner is the person with the least number of stickers on them at the end.

Direct Speech Work

At the end of the least-first continuum is working directly on the child's speech. In this approach, non-fluency and any associated problems are tackled directly. At this stage, there is an inherent acknowledgement that speech is a problem that requires modification and change. Therefore, attempts are made to decrease the dysfluencies by teaching fluency-enhancing techniques.

The following are some techniques which could be taught to the child when adopting this approach.

Easy onset

This technique is useful especially if the child is experiencing difficulty initiating speech. Easy onset, once mastered, allows some control over 'starting off', which often then gives non-fluent speakers the confidence to proceed with the rest of the utterance.

This technique takes the main processes of voice production – respiration and phonation – and separates them into two phases. It can be described to clients as a technique which simplifies the process of initiating speech by getting one process going before starting the next.

Respiration phase First, speakers are taught normal breathing for speech, that is, short inhalation with extended, controlled exhalation. A relaxed posture and approach is encouraged. Then clients move into exhalation, with anticipated speech production following. (Some clients find it useful to position their articulators for the initial sound while exhaling.) The clinician models inhalation, then exhalation, of a small amount of air. Clients should be encouraged to produce a relaxed air flow and not blow the air out. Once clients are successful at this process, the phonation phase can be introduced.

Phonation phase The fundamental principle of this phase is the gradual onset of voicing, accompanied by light articulatory contacts. After air flow has commenced, clients are taught to 'slide' slowly into the first sound, slightly increasing the time taken to articulate the sound. The remainder of the word is completed in a normal way. (Some clients have a tendency to use a rising inflection when producing this first sound in a gradual manner. This is usually eliminated as the individual becomes more proficient in the use of the technique.)

We recommend that clinicians teach this technique using vowels, semi-vowels/liquids and continuants in the first instance. Plosives are best saved until last, as some distortion of sound is inevitable when at this stage the plosive phase is slowed down during practice.

Children can be taught the technique principally through modelling by the clinician. Once they are able to demonstrate the technique on isolated sounds, the following structured approach can be used to achieve production in spontaneous speech:

- *CV/VC monosyllabic level.* Practise the technique on initial English consonants (C) and vowels (V). (With children, we use graphemes rather than phonemes, even though this means duplication of some sounds, such as /k/ and omitting others, such as /tʃ/.)
- *Phrase level.* Here, clients are encouraged to practise easy onset at the beginning of short two-, three- and four-word phrases (for example, an apple, a green apple, a green apple tree). This practice can be carried out by reading the phrases. However, we find it more useful to work on spontaneous speech as soon as practicable.
- *Spontaneous speech practice – one-word level.* The clinician may present 'mastermind' type questions requiring a single-word response, with an easy onset at the beginning of the word. For example:
  - What is the capital of France?
  - What is two plus three?
  - What is the name/number of your house?
  - What is your best friend called?
  - Tell me one thing you have in your pocket.
- *Spontaneous speech practice – two- or three-word phrases.* When working at this level, there is a tendency to elicit lists rather than connected sentences.

Lists may be an appropriate first step, but the clinician should move on to related sentences as soon as possible. Examples for these two steps:

– Lists

Tell me three things a monster might have in his home.

What three things might a fireman do when he was fighting a fire?

Ask me three things about my home.

– Related sentences

Tell me how to draw a man/woman.

Describe how you get to your school.

Tell me about your favourite character from a book/film/cartoon.

◆ *Continuous speech.* The aim of working at this level is to enable the child to use easy onset at the beginning of any breath group and/or at any time when he anticipates a non-fluency occurring. To that end, we work first with reading passages and then with spontaneous speech. One activity which we have used successfully with both is 'token surprise'.

Token surprise: the clinician has a supply of coloured tokens or Smarties on the desk in front of the child. During a reading activity, a monologue or conversation, the clinician will place one token in the child's line of vision. This will indicate to the child that he is to start the next word with an easy onset.

The clinician should vary the initial phonemes and the position in the sentence.

Once children are proficient at such activities, they should be encouraged to use the easy onset technique when they are dysfluent and when they anticipate difficulty. With some children it may be necessary to carry out transfer activities. In this case, a hierarchy of situations of increasing difficulty will be agreed with the child and worked through in a systematic way. An example of such a hierarchy follows:

◆ At home with the dog

◆ At home with my Mum

◆ At home when talking with the family over breakfast

◆ When walking to school with my best friend

◆ At school during break with my best friend and one or two other classmates

◆ At school talking to a group of friends at lunch time

- In class when working in small groups
- Answering the teacher when by myself
- Answering the teacher when with my best friend
- Answering the teacher when working in small groups in class
- Answering the teacher when there are several of my friends listening
- Answering an easy question in front of the class
- Answering a difficult question in front of the class.

Using appropriate contrasts: smooth and bumpy

A useful concept to help children understand how and what to change in their speech is the notion of smooth and bumpy talking. A number of commercially available programmes have used this to good effect. The Myers & Woodford (1992) programme uses puppets (racehorse and turtle) to convey the difference and, more recently, Snooky the Snail has been used in a similar way.

The basic idea is the contrast between speech which is 'smooth' and that which creates dysfluency or 'bumps'. In our work, we adapt the information we give to the child (and parent/carer) according to the nature of the child's speaking difficulties. If, for example, we think the child would be helped by reducing his speech rate, then we would include that in our description of what 'smooth' is like.

These appropriate contrasts are then used by the clinician, with the child listening out for errors, including 'bumps'. Later on, roles are reversed and the child is encouraged to use this new pattern in utterances of gradually increasing length.

Speech rate

1 *Observing rate.* A good way of understanding how slowly/quickly people talk is to observe a person such as a newsreader. Children may opt to observe a well-known person from children's television. They need to be given help to notice a number of features associated with rate:

   (a) Number of pauses

   (b) Where the pausing occurs

(c) Pausing for breath

(d) Pausing for dramatic effect and/or emphasis

(e) Rate of some words and phrases in relation to others (that is, the uneven pace of utterances).

2 *Identify and experiment with rate.* Children can be encouraged to change their own rate firstly through experimentation. A clinician may help by timing a set number of words or syllables and then getting the child to increase or decrease the time taken. Discussions then take place to identify how the child was able to achieve both the increased and the slower rate. Alternatively, the child can experiment with saying more or fewer words or syllables within a set time. Again, the important issue for the child is to identify what helps to reduce and increase their utterance length. Examples include:

(a) Taking more time to breathe

(b) Pausing at phrase junctures

(c) Not starting speech immediately

(d) Taking more time over individual articulatory contacts.

3 *Situational hierarchy.* The child may next use a hierarchy to identify situations which can be said at a normal rate, slow rate or fast rate. We have found that introducing the notion of using gears/braking in a car is useful in getting children to understand the dynamic nature of speech rate.

Soft articulatory contacts

This was included at an earlier level, but here, at the point of working directly on children's speech, the focus is on production rather than observation, listening and discrimination. As with all tasks with children, it is important to make speech activities fun. Discussing articulation, pressure and muscle tension is a recipe for switching children off if it is not 'dressed up' in some acceptable fashion. We have used puppets, toys and any current television or cartoon character to get children interested in this particular area. (We note that the Swindon Fluency Packs [McNeil *et al*, 2003] use the same technique.) So tasks in this area may feature Mr Slide or Miss Gentle, or in some cases Sophie the Softie and Bobby the Bumper to explain the contrasts of hard and soft attack. Similarly, articulators can be given names if the children are young.

We would use these characters firstly to help the children identify the difference between a hard and soft articulatory contact in the therapist's production. This starts at isolated sound level, and will progress to the beginning sound of a sentence. The roles are then reversed, and the children are required to produce the appropriate contact for the character in question (for example, 'Sophie or Bobby sitting on your lips'), first in isolation, then at the beginning of monosyllabic words, polysyllabic words, and short phrases, and then to begin sentences.

An example of a progression of an activity using these characters is as follows. First (Table 9) many of the more easily identifiable speech sounds would be introduced and the child encouraged to say the sound with both a hard and soft contact:

Table 9 Sophie the Softie and Bobby the Bumper as aids in saying sounds		
What to say	Use Sophie the Softie	Use Bobby the Bumper
Lip sounds	P,P,P,P,P,P	P,P,P,P,P,P
	B,B,B,B,B,	B,B,B,B,B
	W,W,W,W,W	W,W,W,W,W
Lip & teeth sounds	F,F,F,F,F	F,F,F,F,F
	V,V,V,V,V	V,V,V,V,V
Tongue sounds	L,L,L,L,L	L,L,L,L,L
	S,S,S,S,S	S,S,S,S,S
	Z,Z,Z,Z,Z	Z,Z,Z,Z,Z
	T,T,T,T,T	T,T,T,T,T
	D,D,D,D,D	D,D,D,D,D
	K,K,K,K,K	K,K,K,K,K
	G,G,G,G,G	G,G,G,G,G
'Nosey' sounds	M,M,M,M,M	M,M,M,M,M
	N,N,N,N,N	N,N,N,N,N
'Open' sounds	A,A,A,A,A	A,A,A,A,A
	EE,EE,EE,EE,EE	EE,EE,EE,EE,EE
	OO,OO,OO,OO,OO	OO,OO,OO,OO,OO

Taking the 'lip sounds', the progression may be as shown in Table 10:

Table 10 Sophie the Softie and Bobby the Bumper as aids in the progression of lip sounds		
Lip Sounds: **What to say**	**Use Sophie the Softie**	**Use Bobby the Bumper**
Short words	PEA POOH PIE BEE BOW BAR	PEA POOH PIE BEE BOW BAR
Longer words	PETAL PUDDLE BOTTLE BUMPER	PETAL PUDDLE BOTTLE BUMPER
Phrases	PLEASE CAN I? PENNIES TO SPEND BUT WHY NOT BLUE IS FOR ME	PLEASE CAN I? PENNIES TO SPEND BUT WHY NOT BLUE IS FOR ME
Sentences	PAMELA IS MY FRIEND'S NAME POOH BEAR EATS HONEY BOYS LIKE TO KICK STONES BLACKBIRDS ARE IN MY GARDEN	PAMELA IS MY FRIEND'S NAME POOH BEAR EATS HONEY BOYS LIKE TO KICK STONES BLACKBIRDS ARE IN MY GARDEN

Relaxation Techniques

We have learnt through several difficult experiences how *not* to work on relaxation with children. Many do not respond well to the quiet, calming activities that can be very effective with adults. Relaxation for most children needs to be an active, doing process in which they experience positive contrasts and/or engage in behaviours during which relaxation is a significant by-product.

1 **Contrasts – general movements.** Children are encouraged to adopt the stance and/or movements of the following. It is important to keep the sequence or appropriate order to ensure the contrast of tense/relaxed:

   (a) Clown – robot figure

   (b) Rag doll – giant with heavy boots

   (c) Jack-in-the-box on wobbly spring – knight in full armour

   (d) Someone sunbathing on a very hot day – someone trying to keep warm outside on a very frosty winter's day

   (e) Carefree child – marching soldier.

2 **Contrasts – specific movements.** Clinicians may need to model these specific muscle contrasts before children will grasp what is required. Examples include:

   (a) Tense fingers by clenching or fanning out and then relax/flop

   (b) Tense toes by clenching or fanning out and then relax/flop

   (c) Tense shoulders by lifting to ears or pushing down to floor and then relax

   (d) Tense stomach by pulling in towards back and then relax

   (e) Tense face by scrunching up whole face or stretching mouth wide and opening eyes wide and then letting go.

   Each exercise should be repeated up to five times.

   In addition, there are a number of texts which detail more extensive programmes for the development of relaxation with children, for example *Relax and Be Happy* (Madders, 1987), *Relaxation for Children* (Rickard, 1996).

3 Reading, playing games, building an object, and doing a jigsaw are all activities in which many children can engage, and experience relaxation as a by-product. If these activities are suggested, care must be taken to ensure that any stressors, such as time pressure, the element of competition and so on, are removed.

Central or Diaphragmatic Breathing

In our experience, teaching children to change their breathing patterns is very difficult. We have tried it with children of 9/10 years of age, and feel that the end result was far from satisfactory.

With these younger children, we believe that it is enough to convey the rudiments of exhalation/inhalation and speaking on an outward breath stream. This can be discussed using balloons and games involving extended exhalation time. (See Chapter 8 on group therapy for specific examples.)

With older children, it is again advisable to engage them in an activity that demonstrates the process, rather than discussing the process in a more theoretical manner. We have had some success with children lying on their backs and placing a book on their diaphragm to give them the idea of a central breathing pattern. Similarly, observing clavicular movements in a full-length mirror can be the first step to inhibiting these extraneous movements and developing a more relaxed breathing pattern.

In both cases, there should be a move, early in therapy, towards using this more efficient breathing pattern in speech. Once again, we would approach this by giving children activities which require gradually increasing lengths of utterance.

The Lidcombe Programme

Perhaps one of the greatest influences on the treatment of stammering in young children in the past few years has been the development of the Lidcombe Programme originating from Australia.

The Lidcombe Programme is described as 'an operant treatment for early stuttering that is presented by parents in children's everyday environments' (Packman & Onslow, 2000, p267). Stammering is seen essentially as a speech problem that children need to learn to manage in all areas of their life, rather than in an altered environment (Onslow & Packman, 1999). The authors accept that, during therapy, changes are made to the child's environment, but this is in order that the programme can be best presented to the child, rather than because of a belief that factors in the environment are responsible for the child's stammering. The principle behind therapy is that reinforcing fluent speech will lead to more fluency, whereas 'correction' of dysfluency will lead the child to decrease the behaviour. The aim of therapy is to help the child become consistently stammer-free, initially in practice sessions, and then to generalise the fluency to all situations. The programme is said to be conceptually simple but procedurally complex. Packman & Onslow (2000, p268) noted that one major difference between this approach and others is that 'it is presented by parents where the problem occurs, namely, in the child's everyday environment'. Essentially, the clinician's role is to teach parents to carry out the treatment at home and to problem-solve with them. Parents give feedback to the child ('verbal response contingent stimulation') in response to both fluent and dysfluent speech ('smooth' and 'bumpy' talking), with the emphasis on praise for smooth talking initially and some more limited 'correction' of bumpy talking as treatment progresses. The clinician teaches the parent how to carry out structured sessions at home and, once these have been successfully established, feedback is introduced into unstructured everyday speaking situations. Once the child has achieved low ratings for stammering severity in these sessions, they enter the next phase of therapy in which the parent gradually withdraws feedback.

Measurement is seen as an integral part of the therapy process. Two kinds of measures are carried out, one by the clinician, the other by the parent. The clinician uses a 'percentage syllables stuttered' measure, taken from 300 syllables of the child's conversational speech at the clinic visits (visits are initially weekly and increasingly less often in the maintenance phase). The parent carries out daily measurements using a 10-point severity scale, in which a score of 1 indicates no stuttering and a score of 10 indicates extremely severe stuttering.

Therapy is carefully structured, and sessions are manipulated in order that the child achieves a high degree of success and activities are fun for both child and parent. Therapy is individualised for each particular child.

Research into the Lidcombe Programme

Various studies carried out into the effectiveness of the Lidcombe Programme have yielded encouraging results; however, at the time of writing, the results of a randomised control trial have not been published. The Australian Stuttering Research Centre web site (www3.fhs.usyd.edu.au/asrcwww/treatment/lidcombe.htm) summarises research so far.

The Lidcombe Programme is now widely used in the UK and for some clinicians here, as for many in Australia, it is used as the initial approach with all young stammering children. For others, it is part of a 'package' of approaches, often not used unless less direct interventions have failed to produce desired change. Some clinicians are also experimenting with a variety of ways of delivering the approach, in response to practical obstacles of more conventional delivery (for example, parents unable to attend because of work commitments). Williams & Whitehead (2002) have, for example, trialled what they describe as a successful adapted form of programme delivery. This starts with an intensive day's training for parents and children, followed by phone contact, audiotaped data and monthly reviews.

Many criticisms have been raised against the programme, and we ourselves were initially very uneasy about it. We still rarely use it as a first approach, preferring the 'least first' approach. We have not found Lidcombe to work for everyone and for some families, however highly motivated and keen to help their child, the complications of family life can make the availability of even 10 minutes of individual time for one parent and one child well-nigh impossible. We have noted that its use can also be problematic for children who find its structure limiting, for example, talkative children who want to tell you all they know about something in response to 'What is this?' when a one-word answer is what is required. These and other problems, however, can often be resolved when the problem-solving approach advocated by the Lidcombe Programme is adopted.

Perhaps one of the strongest fears expressed has been that drawing attention to a young child's stammering will increase the stammering, either overtly or, perhaps more worryingly, covertly. Certainly, attitudes towards openness around stammering have changed considerably over the past decades. A study by Woods *et al* (2002) revealed that there were no systemic negative effects (such as anxiety, aggression, withdrawal or depression) associated with the use of the programme, and Woods *et al* (2002, p37) concluded that there is 'no reason to doubt that the Lidcombe Programme of early stuttering intervention is a safe treatment'.

The Lidcombe Programme is essentially a parental programme. It can be extremely empowering for a parent to feel that they have been instrumental in bringing fluency to their child. Equally, if the child does not achieve the hoped-for changes, it is quite likely that a parent may take responsibility for the failure. Clearly, therapists need to be sensitive to this possibility.

In conclusion, our view is currently that the Lidcombe Programme has a lot to offer many children and families. We personally do not see it as the first therapeutic approach that we would use with a young stammering child, and still prefer to work initially with parents on a wide range of communication and environmental issues and sometimes giving the child the experience of controlling their own fluency. We prefer to start with less time-consuming, less 'hands-on' methods and use Lidcombe if these approaches have not had the desired outcomes. We believe the Lidcombe Programme to be inappropriate with some families because of their circumstances, lifestyle or lack of problem-solving skills.

Therapists using the approach in Britain would benefit from the regular updates, discussions and support mechanisms that are commonplace in Australia. We also need to compare the way therapists in the two countries are using the approach so that our outcomes can be fairly compared. It may be that we are selecting clients differently (for example it seems that Australian therapists may wait until a child is 12 months post onset of stammering before commencing the Lidcombe Programme, and only assessment and monitoring take place until then). Perhaps the programme is applied differently in the two countries (for example, in the way severity ratings are applied or levels of language output monitored). We will continue to learn more about these similarities and differences and the Programme will continue to be modified and developed in the light of research and clinical observation. We have no doubt that the Lidcombe Programme should be a part of the repertoire of any clinician working with stammering in young children.

SUMMARY

We have chosen three therapy options on the least first continuum purposely, as they perhaps represent three distinct points at which there is a change of approach. In reality, there may be considerable overlap, with the clinician choosing an approach at any point along that continuum depending upon her evaluation of the child's needs. By looking at the various disadvantages and advantages, a therapist can evaluate what is to be gained by the chosen therapy option, and what may be lost. We know that clinicians do consider their intervention carefully, but with this group of clients especially, therapy has to be the difference which, as a minimum, maintains the status quo and, at best, tips the scales in favour of fluency.

Chapter 7: Confirmed Stammering

DEFINITION

The words 'confirmed stammering' appear at first sight to contain little hope. If something is confirmed, surely it is final and not open to change? We take the view that, whilst this final stage in the development of stammering is of concern, it is not as final as its description implies. We take heart from Kelly's optimistic view of the world, which sees change as always possible:

> 'We take the stand that there are always some alternative constructions available to choose among in dealing with the world. No one needs to paint himself into a corner; no one needs to be completely hemmed in by circumstances; no one needs to be a victim of his own biography.' (1991, p11)

So what do we mean when we use the term 'confirmed stammerer'? Once again, we feel the key is in children's construing of their dysfluency, in our so-called fifth dimension. Children or young people who we feel fit this category construe themselves as stammerers, regardless of the severity or otherwise of their overt symptoms, and use certain behaviours in order to hide or deny the stammer. We do not suggest a specific age band for this stage of development, as we are only too aware that it can on occasions be seen in children of primary school age or, conversely, be absent in adulthood. However, as the majority of young people we see who have reached this stage are in the teenage years, we will refer to this age group in our explanations and examples. Once again we refer to our five dimensions, this time to describe confirmed stammering:

1 **Quantitative.** Although it is commonly the case that overt symptoms increase in quantity, both in terms of total stammering and in number of iterations, another common scenario is for the amount of stammering actually to decrease as individuals find more ways in which to hide their stammering. The stammer can also start to be more apparent in particular situations, as children begin to anticipate stammering (or not stammering) in particular situations or to construe situations differently in terms of fear of stammering.

2 **Qualitative.** Peters & Guitar (1991, p97) characterise the core stammering behaviours of 'intermediate stammerers' as blocks, which they describe as

occurring in one or more of three ways: 'stopping airflow, voicing or movement'. This is followed by a struggle to restart. Other behaviours, such as word and sound repetitions with multiple iterations, and prolongations, may also be apparent as children increase their efforts to do something about their speech. SLDs may stay at much the same level or even increase, with iterations becoming more rapid in some cases.

3 **Physical.** Struggle behaviour is likely to be apparent in overt speech behaviours. Many of the behaviours seen in borderline stammering may be evident and magnified.

4 **Physiological.** Concomitant movements may develop or increase during this stage, as young people strive to reduce their overt stammering. They may tap their feet while talking or clench their fists. They may act on the advice of others and take a deep breath before a difficult word. These actions may temporarily increase fluency, but too often, of course, the positive effect is short-lived but the habit becomes incorporated as part of the stammer. Some concomitant movements can serve to hide from the individual those reactions they do not want to see, for example, if they look away from the listener or close their eyes they cannot see their listener's embarrassment. Other behaviours are part of the embarrassment they themselves are feeling, such as blushing or sometimes giggling. So what we see at this stage is a 'confirmation' of these behaviours as part of the whole picture of stammering.

5 **Psychological.** The greatest change associated with young people's stammering is likely to occur in relation to avoidance behaviours. Young people with confirmed stammers try to hide their stammering in a variety of ways. Some of these avoidances may be more obvious to a tuned-in listener; others may be more subtle, and some almost impossible to spot. Word avoidance may be cleverly disguised, not only by substitution but by fillers, feigning forgetfulness or thinking time, using postponement devices, leaving sentences unfinished, circumlocution and so on. Situation avoidance, too, may develop. Young people may no longer be prepared to run errands, may go to their rooms as soon as they come in from school, play incessantly on the

computer and refuse to call on friends. Of course, these behaviours are not uncommon in any number of non-stammering adolescents, which makes our task of understanding how much the stammer is responsible for the actions all the more difficult. Young people can also become very adroit at concealing their stammers and adopt quite sophisticated strategies to ensure that others do not become aware of the problem. Among the features of confirmed stammering are the anticipation and construing of stammering, as we will see later.

THE ADOLESCENT WHO STAMMERS

Let us now turn to look at adolescents who, in addition to all the difficulties which this stage of development brings, also stammer. We noted earlier that one of the most important changes that occurs in confirmed stammering is in the person's construing. This is the area we will now examine.

Construing of Stammering

For us, the most important clue to whether a young person is becoming a confirmed stammerer is in the way he construes the problem. If his stammer is seen as frustrating or an inconvenience but does not prevent him from feeling generally positive about his speaking ability, we would regard it as borderline, rather than confirmed. If, however, he has progressed from a stage of fleeting awareness and has a view of himself now negatively coloured by his dysfluency, then he is likely to have reached this further stage. The behaviours already outlined above will help form a picture of the meaning of the stammer to an individual. The following are some suggestions of other areas to explore in trying to complete the picture:

◆ Does the young person construe himself in terms of stammering? Does he construe himself, in speaking situations, more in terms of how he speaks than what he says? If he makes an interesting contribution but stammers, does he feel a greater sense of achievement than if he said something of no great import but remained fluent?

- Does he construe other people or other situations in terms of his own stammering behaviour? 'He makes me stammer/he doesn't'; 'I always stammer at his house/I never stammer at hers'.

- Does he believe that others construe him predominantly in terms of his stammer? Is the stammer the part he thinks others are most aware of/concerned about?

- Does he make decisions that appear to be based on stammering? For example, does he choose hobbies which do not demand verbal interaction? Does he make friends with outgoing people who are happy to do all the talking, or quiet people who demand little of him? Does he make subject choices at school that demand little speaking, and give up as soon as possible those which demand more?

- Does he blame his stammer for his poor performance? ('If I didn't stammer I'd be the best at French'; 'I'm a much better reader than the rest of the class, but they don't know because I always stammer on long words'.)

- Does he appear to have a sense of resignation about his speech, a feeling that whatever he or anyone else does, nothing will change?

- Does he have a 'don't care' attitude to his stammer or deny that it concerns him in any way, when the evidence suggests otherwise?

- Is he a loner? Does he keep his feelings to himself or, conversely, does he become easily aggressive? Might any of these behaviours suggest that he is trying to avoid being hurt or to else be used to gain some control over how he allows his stammer to affect him?

- Does he seem to construe himself as different from others; does he feel/appear out of place with his peer group?

Techniques for understanding

Personal construct therapists have offered a number of ideas to help workers understand children's construing. Many of the techniques described below will also be appropriate for use with borderline stammering, but are outlined together here for reasons of clarity.

Using repertory grids The way in which these are completed will vary according to the age and maturity of the child. Some will be able to follow the adult format for elicitation of constructs and elements and for rating. With others, the completion of a grid may not be appropriate or possible. Yet others can complete the task using a much simplified process. Hayhow & Levy (1989) offer a number of suggestions as to how to do this.

Kelly's (1991) self-characterisation This can be used in its original form as a way of helping older or more mature children express how they see themselves. Jackson describes an alternative format for use with younger or less mature children:

> Tell me what sort of boy or girl [name] is. If you like I will be your secretary and write down what you say. Tell me about yourself as if you were being described by an imaginary friend who knows you well and likes you and above all understands you very well. This person would be able to say what your character is and everything about you. Perhaps you could begin with [*Name*] *is* ... and say something important about yourself. Try to fill this page. (1988, p224)

Jackson (1988) suggested a way of analysing self-characterisations along personal construct psychology lines, based around the corollaries to the fundamental postulate expounded in Kelly's work (1991). A brief outline of these is given below, with possible examples:

1   **View of others** (sociality corollary). References to the way the child sees other people as construing him (for example, 'His mum says he's untidy').

2   **Personal history and future** (experience corollary). References made by the child to his own past or future, in psychological terms (for example, 'He used to be good at football').

3   **Psychological cause and effect** (construction corollary). References made in terms of cause and effect. These may be explicit (for example, 'He's lazy because he always leaves things to the last minute') or implicit ('He is helpful. He clears away after breakfast').

4   **Non-psychological statements** (dichotomy corollary). Physical descriptions or statements of behaviours or activities (for example, 'He goes to high school').

5   **Psychological statements** (organisation corollary). Any statements made that have a psychological component (for example, 'She hates doing her piano practice').

6   **Contradictions** (fragmentation corollary). Remarks or themes that are contradictory ('He has lots of friends'; 'He is often alone at break').

7   **Insight** (choice corollary). The child's awareness of his own shortcomings/problems ('She is always falling out with her best friend').

8   **Self-esteem** (individuality and commonality corollaries). Claims of competence ('She's a good speller') or of moral virtue ('He is never bored').

Self-characterisations can help us to try to enter into children's developing construct systems and to understand the way in which children are attempting to make sense of their world.

Ravenette's techniques   A variety of techniques offered by Ravenette can be used to further a therapist's understanding. Although these references may seem dated, we still find the material extremely powerful and relevant.

1   **Elaboration of complaints** (Ravenette, 1977, p270). The focus of this technique is described as 'the complaints which an individual voices against people who might be important in his life'). Children's construing of some of the difficulties they may be experiencing can be explored, and possible solutions or alternatives considered.

2   **Perceptions of troubles in school** (Ravenette, 1977). Eight rather vague pictures of school events are presented and children are invited to choose the person who is troubled, and then are asked various questions. Ravenette suggested that the responses can help the clinician to ascertain how children view and identify with the situations, the variety of ways in which they may deal with them and possibilities for change.

3   Portrait gallery (Ravenette, 1980). Drawings of two schematic faces are used to show a sad and a happy child. Children are first asked which is sad and which is happy, and then to say three things about each. Other blank faces are presented for children to fill in according to a variety of other ways they identify a child as feeling. Using such a technique can help children to identify and amplify some of the emotions they experience.

4   The good and bad of it (Ravenette, 1980). Children are helped to identify 'problems' they are experiencing and then are asked to look at both the bad and the good things about it. Ravenette suggested that such an exploration can help children look at some of the implications of the problem and the possible obstacles to change. A child who stammers may, for example, state 'I always cry when my brother laughs at me for stammering'. The bad thing about this may be that the child feels bad, but the good thing may be that the brother gets punished.

Genograms   Hayhow & Levy (1989) suggested the use of genograms (family trees) in which the child (with or without the aid of parents) can pictorially illustrate his family and can be encouraged to examine relationships between family members. Our experience of the use of genograms in a group of adolescents proved to be an enjoyable activity for the young people and gave the clinicians certain insights that they may not have otherwise had. This is described further in Chapter 9.

Ravenette (1977) pointed to the relevance of this style of interviewing for the child, referring to it as a 'stocktaking or a mapping exercise' (p279) through which children are helped to be more aware of how they are currently making sense of the world and, it is hoped, becoming open to experimenting with alternative constructions.

Who Am I?   (Nightingale, 1986) This publication contains photocopiable sheets aimed at helping adolescents to understand themselves and the ways in which they relate to others. It explores many of the issues with which this age group are particularly concerned (appearance, friendships, relationships with parents and so on). We have found these a useful basis for discussion, both with individuals and with groups.

Psychodrama This can be a very powerful way of working with children's feelings. We have been very fortunate to work with Gail Smith, who is, to our knowledge, the only British Speech & Language Therapist working in the NHS who is trained in this method. We cannot begin to work in as skilled and complete a way as our colleague, but we have been able to refer children to her to work with in this powerful way, both individually and in groups. She has also introduced us to some techniques that we have been able to use ourselves and have found very useful:

Doubling Smith (2002, p63) described the two functions of this technique as 'emotional holding and stretching of the protagonist's internal world'. Bannister (2002, pp22–23) outlined how 'a member of the therapeutic group comes alongside the protagonist (or key player in the drama) and copies their movements or bodily position and also endeavours to vocalise the feelings. The protagonist may accept or reject the words of the "double", but it is important that the position of the body, or expression of the face, expresses the true feeling more accurately than the spoken word.' We have found this a most helpful technique to show children how we are really trying to be empathic and to understand what they are feeling but may or may not feel able to express. Smith (personal communication, March 2004), has told us that she finds doubling of particular value with children who may present with some resistance or fear of participating in therapy. She believes that the technique of doubling allows a clinician metaphorically to step out of their own role into an aspect of a child's internal world.

Role reversal This technique helps children to explore and understand the way another person may be feeling. Smith (2002) gave the example of *T* who was asked to step into the role of her English teacher and see the teacher's attitude towards *T*'s stammer in a different way, perhaps challenging her own previous perception.

Mirroring Bannister (2002, p23) described this technique in which 'the adult repeats the words and actions of the child so that they can see how they are perceived by others'. She stressed the need to do this in a supportive way.

INTERVENTION WITH THE CONFIRMED STAMMERER

Many therapists view the treatment of young people in this stage of stammering development with some trepidation. The 'what if?' feeling (what if he stammers when he goes to school/when he gets married/goes for an interview?) that so often worries parents of even very young dysfluent children can now begin to be a focus of concern for the clinician, who knows how debilitating a problem stammering can be in adulthood. While most would agree that therapy should include consideration of feelings and attitudes, adolescents can be withdrawn and insular and reluctant to talk about these issues. Instead, they may demand techniques that can, in fact, serve to increase the ways they already have for hiding the stammering behaviour. They often resist any suggestions aimed to help them become more open about stammering, seeing very little of relevance in this kind of approach.

So what should we be aiming to achieve in our therapy with this group? Below are some general principles which we feel should be taken into account. We must always bear in mind that each person we work with is an individual and, as such, has individual needs.

Help the Client to Reconstrue

We have stated that one of the most important factors in this stage of development is young people's construing of themselves as stammerers and their construing of other people and of situations in terms of a stammering role. Therefore one of the underlying principles in our therapy should be to help our clients to reconstrue themselves, others, stammering and situations in which they communicate, in a more positive way. We aim to return our clients to the early stage of development, where the stammer was concerned with speech production but did not carry a host of other implications.

Reconstruing self

Clients can be helped to look at themselves in other ways than as people who stammer. Elaboration of personal qualities can enhance self-esteem and help them construe themselves along dimensions other than stammering-fluent. Experiments can be constructed in which the young people rate themselves along a number of dimensions that they see as important in others but only useful for themselves as secondary to stammering. *S*, for example, discovered that, when he gave a talk at school, even though he stammered, he was actually not only an interesting speaker, but came across as a better communicator than many of his fluent peers.

Reconstruing listener reactions

Adolescents are particularly sensitive to how they are seen by others. We have only to recall how the smallest of spots can make an attractive teenager feel he has turned into Frankenstein's monster, to realise how true this is! Observation exercises can help adolescents understand that stammering is only one of a large number of ways in which others form opinions of them. Listener reactions to stammering are often perceived as negative, regardless of whether there is any concrete evidence that this is actually the case. *B* made up any number of reasons for leaving school early in order to go to speech therapy; the fear of her friends' reactions to the 'truth' was so great. It had not dawned on her for an instant that there were alternative ways in which her friends might react – for example, with interest, curiosity or even admiration. Surveys on stammering (see Chapter 10) can help shift clients' perceptions of how others see stammering.

Reconstruing stammering

Stammering is not only nearly always construed negatively but also commonly construed as something the person *is*, rather than something he *does*. Manning (2001, p290) pointed out the implications for maintenance if this aspect of therapy is omitted: 'The client who retains self-defeating mental images and negative thoughts and beliefs about speech and his ability to manage it is much less apt to succeed once he is on his own.' If young confirmed stammerers can be helped to separate the stammer from the core of their construing about themselves, then its implications in all aspects of their lives may be reduced. Understanding the development of stammering can aid this process and free clients from 'taking the blame' for their stammers. Levy (1987) suggested that desensitisation is a synonym for reconstruing stammering. Included here, therefore, are activities aimed to reduce the negative emotions connected with stammering and to toughen young people to the stammer and to negative reactions. Some of these techniques are described later in this chapter. For a fuller explanation readers are referred to Van Riper (1973), Levy (1987) and Reid (1987).

Reconstruing situations

People with confirmed stammers very often construe situations in terms of their stammering behaviour. They may ask themselves if they will have to speak and, if so, whether they have to say any 'difficult' words. This can affect all aspects of their lives – home, friendships, and school. For some young people, bringing this to conscious awareness can help them to confront their stammering and to begin the process of change. For others, looking to the future does not seem relevant, much as telling a young smoker that he could die of cancer or heart disease frequently does not affect his habit. Often, young people do not test out the reality of their predictions, and therapy can help them do so. They may find, eg, that if they answer questions in class there are a range of possible options other than their own firmly held belief that classmates will laugh. They may, in fact, not stammer at all; they may stammer, but receive a favourable reaction or be rewarded for an interesting contribution. One of our clients realised that it was her own laughter at her stammer when speaking in class that led to the laughter of others. When she experimented with reacting calmly and just carrying on after stammering she discovered that her classmates continued to listen. Helping clients consider possible reactions may alert them to alternative possibilities and persuade them to experiment with changing their behaviour. The threat of experimentation must not, however, be too great for the individual concerned and it is important that clients and therapists initially design experiments together, to make sure that results are most likely to be a positive learning experience.

Encouraging Openness

As we have mentioned, one of the most important changes that occurs between borderline and confirmed stammering is the tendency to hide the stammer. This can create a vicious circle – increasing feelings that the stammer is bad and must not be revealed at all costs. Helping young people to confront the stammer, to talk about it with those with whom they feel safest, and to let people know that they are going for speech and language therapy can help to break the circle and reduce these negative feelings. Often, people who stammer expect others to be mind readers and to understand their fears and anxieties, to know why they are quiet or unresponsive and so on, when in fact they are doing all they can to ensure that others cannot understand.

Once people have talked about the stammer, they are often surprised at how interested the other person is. Often, too, the listener's embarrassment is reduced when he is 'given permission' to notice the stammer, rather than a non-verbal suggestion not to notice at any cost! Talking about the stammer also allows an individual to tell the listener how they would like them to respond, rather than letting the listener do what he thinks may be best, but which might in fact be unhelpful.

Sometimes young people amaze us in their ability to be open about their stammering. One of our clients, for example, chose to do his final year project at primary school on stammering, including in it interviews with his friend, his father (who also stammers) and his clinician. He was also happy for us to share it with other young people. Another took an active part in a presentation on stammering that we gave to her class. Others have chosen stammering as their topic for a class talk or have designed leaflets for their teachers, to inform them about stammering in general and as it relates to them as individuals.

The very process of understanding more about stammering can help some young people to feel a greater sense of control. Using a leaflet such as *Teenagers and Young Adults who Stammer* (British Stammering Association [BSA]) can help to open up the subject, answer questions that young people may have found difficult to ask and give practical ideas and strategies. We have also found the book *Do you Stutter: A Guide for Teens* (Fraser & Perkins, 2000) to be a useful way of opening up communication. We often suggest that clients read one or two of these easy and short chapters between sessions and bring back points raised which do and do not apply to them for discussion in the next session.

We have found various videos to be useful in part or as an entirety. The BSA has various ones that can be borrowed. *The School-Age Child who Stutters* (Stuttering

Foundation of America) features young people who stammer and well-known clinicians (Barry Guitar, Hugo Gregory and Paul Ramig) in conversation to discuss three areas in particular: what is stammering? (causes, who it affects, variability, what is involved, and so on), feelings and important aspects of self-help and therapy.

Diary writing also gives young people a way of telling us things they can find difficult to mention face-to-face. We have found this to be especially useful with teenage girls.

Reducing Avoidance

Reducing avoidance can be a very frightening process for young people who have maintained a reasonably high level of fluency through avoiding difficult words and situations. It is often hard for them to understand the rationale behind this kind of approach: 'What can be wrong with saying soccer instead of football if it means you can be fluent?'; 'Why answer a question in class if you will stammer and be ridiculed?' Indeed, we have known parents to suggest this very course of action to their offspring as, at face value, it seems to offer a sensible solution. We would therefore suggest that it is of prime importance that young people and those involved with them fully understand the reasoning behind avoidance reduction and the long-term effects that this can produce. It is important that we make such explanations relevant to the particular young person; for example, for a Leeds United fan to avoid the word 'Leeds' and even feel forced to pretend to support a different team could be traumatic! It is also necessary to guard against an elimination of avoidance 'at a stroke'. The increase in dysfluency that this may produce can be catastrophic and only serve to convince clients that avoidance is the best solution.

We therefore suggest working on avoidance in small steps. Initially, it is helpful for young people to spend some time in identifying occasions on which they avoid and the nature of the avoidance and of the situations, in order to see if there are any patterns. The therapy room itself is an obvious place to commence avoidance reduction, with clients admitting to any attempts to avoid and then saying the feared word over again until any fear is extinguished. Reducing avoidance outside can be instigated using a hierarchy, but this must be designed by the client. This increases a feeling of commitment and control. Once this has been established, clients may be encouraged to actively seek out previously avoided words and situations.

It is often a good idea to carry out avoidance reduction work in a group therapy situation. Sending children out in carefully chosen pairs or threes with a clinician can be a spur to doing something previously unthought of, such as asking for information, directions and so on. This is particularly useful with an age group in which peer pressure can be so influential.

Voluntary Stammering

Clinicians who work with adults know that 'voluntary stammering' is often a very difficult technique to 'sell', but that its use can be a turning point for many. It can be a powerful desensitising experience, showing the individual that they can stammer and remain calm, that listener reactions are usually nowhere near as negative as they thought, and that they are able to reduce many of the fears that accompany stammering. If young people are to be persuaded to try out such a seemingly bizarre idea, then it is essential that the rationale is explained clearly to them. An explanation should also be given to significant others, to ensure that attempts with its use are not sabotaged. It should not usually be introduced too early in therapy, before young people have had the opportunity to talk about some of their feelings around stammering, and perhaps begun to speak about it outside. If it is talked about too soon, clients may well take flight because the threat is too great.

Modelling by the therapist in the clinic, on the phone or in outside situations is an important first step and, for many, will be more than a demonstration and rather a desensitising experience in its own right. The process should be gradually introduced outside (perhaps in the company of the clinician or of another young person who is already using voluntary stammering), initially in non-feared situations and on non-feared words.

In our experience, the use and timing of voluntary stammering must be very carefully considered with this client group. Having said this, it is also important to be aware that some young people are far braver than their clinicians. We recall a young man of 17 to whom we introduced the concept of voluntary stammering. Having explained, demonstrated and practised the technique together, we gingerly asked him how many attempts he might make at using voluntary stammering before his next visit. We expected him to say 'one or two'. In fact he said 50! We raised our dropping jaws and just said that often people chose lower numbers than this but if he felt he could attempt this number that would be great. He did! He went on to do talks about his forthcoming gap year to large groups of people, with supreme confidence.

Reducing Struggle Behaviour

We feel that work to reduce the tension in stammering may be a part of therapy for a number of confirmed stammerers. This may take a variety of forms, several of which have already been mentioned in Chapter 6 on borderline stammering. The kind of approach will vary from client to client and will depend to a large degree on the type of stammer – severe or mild, overt or covert, degree of tension involved and the client's attitude to the stammer and willingness to practise. Our concern is that any approach used is compatible with our overall aim of helping the young person to change in a way that will be personally meaningful and can be maintained.

Some clients benefit from work on rate control, finding it easier to gain overall control when speaking at a slower rate. Others may use a technique to help reduce tension or to start a word more easily, such as easy onset or block modification. For those whose intake of breath is reduced or who find exhaling in a controlled way a problem, work on breathing and/or relaxation may be helpful. (For a fuller outline of all of these techniques refer to Turnbull & Stewart, 1999.)

Dealing with Teasing & Bullying

There is no doubt that some children can be very cruel to others who stammer. We feel that we have a variety of roles when looking at this issue with our clients. First, we need to help them to look closely at exactly what is happening by ascertaining the following information:

◆ Is it just one person who is teasing them or several?
◆ Do they have any allies?

◆ How do teachers deal with teasing/bullying, and is there a policy within the school?

◆ Is the person teasing, or merely enquiring in a more or less insensitive way?

◆ How is the child currently dealing with the teasing?

◆ Have they tried out any alternatives? What happened?

Once we feel we have a clear picture of what is happening, we can deal with the situation in a number of ways. Role plays of specific situations with the actual and then a variety of alternative reactions can be a potent way of helping the young person look at alternative courses of action. Most children come up with ideas such as ignoring the teasing, telling a teacher, teasing the child back, or hitting them. It may be necessary to suggest some alternatives that children have not previously thought of, such as admitting the stammering and even mentioning that they are going to therapy, which often takes the wind out of the sails of the teaser. Another approach, illustrated in the video *A Voice in Exile* (Educational Media Film and Video Ltd, 1984) may also be useful for some. The young stammerer concerned, Alan, is mimicked inaccurately. Alan retorts to his oppressor that he has got it wrong: 'You don't say it like that,' he says, and proceeds to repeat the stammered word, stammering in the correct way. Conture (2001, p277) suggested the use of humour to defuse a situation, such as, 'Sometimes my talking will be interrupted due to technical difficulties!'. Although this kind of option, which involves confronting the stammer, often feels too difficult for many children, some, especially older or more mature ones, find it very helpful. *S* found that it enabled him to feel less guilty about stammering when he could acknowledge that it happened but place the blame for teasing on other people's lack of understanding or embarrassment. *P*, on the other hand, had an alternative way of reacting which it was hard to argue with. When asked what he did when teased, he replied that he would either tell the teacher (in which case the other child would get a detention) or would hit the offender. We enquired whether this did not get him into trouble himself. 'Oh no,' said *P*, 'when the teacher finds out why I hit him, he gives him a detention!' Seemingly a 'no lose' situation!

We have found some of our clients to be very inventive in creating responses to those who tease them about their stammering. *N* told someone who teased her, 'You want to be careful you know, it's catching.' *C*'s response to someone who said,

'You can't talk right' was, 'And your point is?'. An idea that comes from children themselves has far more likelihood of being effective.

In more persistent or severe cases of teasing or bullying, it may be necessary for the therapist to consult with the teacher in order to look at possible solutions. We would suggest that such a meeting should take place with the young person present, so that they are involved in any decisions.

We have found the following poem to be very useful for some children in providing a non-verbal means of dealing with teasing, in a rather light-hearted and humorous way:

> **Mart's advice:**
> If somebody's acting big with you,
> if someone's bossing you about,
> look very hard at one of their ears.
> Keep your eyes fixed on it.
> Don't let up.
> Stare at it as if it was
> a mouldy apple.
> Keep staring.
> Don't blink.
> After a bit
> you'll see their hand
> go creeping up to touch it. They're saying to themselves
> 'What's wrong with my ear?'
>
> At that moment
> you know you've won.
>
> Smile.   (*McGough & Rosen*, 1981)

A publication by Stones (1993) entitled *Don't Pick on Me* is written for children themselves to help them to handle bullying. Bullies are defined as 'people who need to hurt, threaten, frighten or control other people' (p8), and are seen as being in need of help as much as their victims. Examples given in the book about the kind of people bullies like to pick on include those with a stammer. Children are encouraged to find their own resources to deal with bullying by recognising their feelings and developing 'inner power' to help them to stick up for themselves. 'Happiness work-outs' are suggested, which may foster the development of positive self-esteem. The advantages and disadvantages of various coping strategies are very sensitively discussed, as are the benefits of confiding in a caring adult. We would highly recommend this book as a basis for discussion, both with clients who may be experiencing these kinds of difficulties and with their parents and teachers.

Palomares & Schilling (2001) looked at ways children can deal with bullying. The book starts by giving information – definitions, profiles, causes, incidence and so on. It is written for an adult reader and outlines ways in which adults can help, eg by raising awareness or by anti-bullying policies. The rest of the book is given over to activities, stories and discussions, to help young people understand more about bullying, express feelings and learn preventative or coping strategies. Photocopiable sheets are designed for each activity.

A company called 'Incentive Plus' also publishes a range of materials in the area of bullying. Their website, www.incentiveplus.co.uk, lists all their varied publications, which include games, videos, guides, books, programmes and manuals.

For further discussion on bullying, see Chapter 10 on working with schools.

Increasing Social & Communication Skills

This area of therapy may be appropriate with young people in the confirmed stage of stammering. For practical ideas, readers should refer to Chapter 6 on borderline stammering.

Rustin *et al* (1994, pp364–5) advocated a holistic 'communications skills approach' when working with adolescents. The theoretical stance for this approach is cognitive behavioural, which 'enables the client to explore the consequences of his or her own actions and the possibilities for change' ... 'the client is empowered to take responsibility for his own progress by actively constructing alternative strategies, by developing hypotheses about the outcome of these strategies, and by being given the opportunity of testing these out.' Their therapy programme has six components – fluency control, relaxation, social skills, problem solving, negotiation and environmental factors.

Problem Solving

If our aim is for young people to maintain the changes they make in therapy, it is necessary to provide them with ways of dealing with future difficulties that may occur. If we provide our clients with answers, they do not develop the tools with which to find their own answers. We feel that, instead, our role should be to help young people to look at ways of approaching difficulties and of discriminating between positive and negative ways of dealing with them. In this way they can feel better equipped to cope by themselves with problems which may occur both during and on termination of therapy.

We use the following approach to problem solving:

1 Define the problem simply

2 Turn the problem into a goal

3 Brainstorm possible solutions (accept any, however outrageous)

4 Discuss advantages and disadvantages of each idea generated

5 Discard impractical, illegal, unworkable ideas

6 Rank order remaining ideas

7 Try out first idea

8 Evaluate and, if one idea has not helped, try the next.

Example

1 Problem: some people laugh when I stammer when I read out in class

2 Formulate a goal

3 Brainstorm ideas (Figure 2)

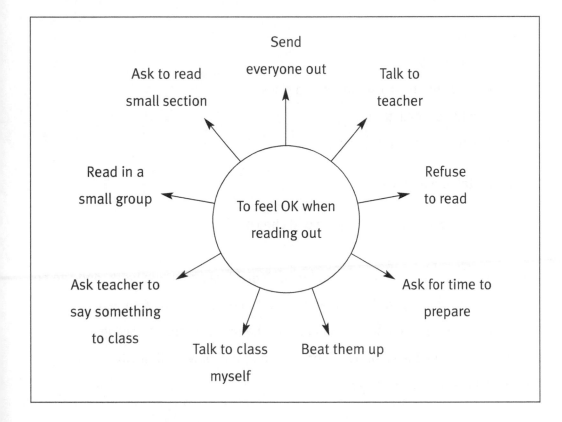

Figure 2 Ideas for brainstorming

4 Advantages and/or disadvantages:

(a) Send everyone out (easier, but not practical)

(b) Talk to teacher (might help, might not)

(c) Refuse to read (would not be allowed)

(d) Ask for time to prepare (just as bad, if not worse)

(e) Beat them up (I'd get in trouble)

(f) Talk to class myself (frightening)

(g) Ask teacher to say something to class (might help, might make it worse)

(h) Read in a small group (easier; teacher may not agree)

(i) Ask to read small section (would be easier, but I might still stammer).

5 Discard ideas:

   (a) Send everyone out

   (b) Refuse to read

   (c) Ask for time to prepare

   (d) Beat them up

   (e) Talk to class myself.

6 Rank order:

   (a) Talk to teacher

   (b) Ask teacher to say something to class

   (c) Read in a small group

   (d) Ask to read small section.

7 Try out talking to teacher.

8 Evaluate and, if necessary, try second choice.

This kind of approach is equally suitable for individual and group work, and can be used both with young people on their own, with their parents or with parents alone. Rustin (1987) gave a number of examples of the use of problem solving in groups, together with some ideas for how therapists might deal with difficulties which may arise when the approach is used.

We have found the publication *Goal* (Grove-Stephenson & Quilliam, 1986) to be a useful resource to use with older children, either individually or in groups, to help them explore alternatives, set goals and consider outcomes.

Reducing Isolation

As we have stated previously, some young people who stammer fear their stammering so much that they will go to great lengths to hide it. This may involve a greater or lesser degree of social isolation. For some, and especially if the person is good at sport or any other participative activity which is not predominantly dependent on speaking, this sense of 'aloneness' may be less apparent. Others develop an interest in hobbies which are solitary, or they just tend to keep to themselves. Often this state of affairs develops without individuals being aware of underlying reasons. Drawing it to conscious attention can help the person realise what is happening and then look at strategies with which to redress the balance. Often, people who stammer have never met anyone else with the same problem. One of the most powerful ways in which a clinician can help to change this picture is by introducing them to others who stammer. This is discussed further in Chapter 8. Helping the young person become more involved socially is another useful strategy. Looking at their interests gives clues to activities, clubs, organisations and extra-curricular activities that they may be interested in joining.

Preparation for 'No Cure'

We believe that this may be a very important function for clinicians in relation to some young confirmed stammerers. Many children have been told for years that they will 'grow out of it', by their parents, friends, medical practitioners and even by clinicians. As they approach adulthood, they must wonder on what authority this well-meant knowledge was based, and why it has not come about. We recall an adult we saw (whose stammer was predominantly covert) telling us that his parents had told him repeatedly that if only he worked hard enough at his speech, all would in due course be well. He did indeed 'work hard' – at hiding it from them and making it appear that they had been right. In reality, the stammer became an integral part of his identity. He learned that it was unacceptable and must not be seen. Along with this determination to hide grew a belief that he was inferior to speakers who did not have this dark secret.

If people's hopes have been focused on a 'cure' for all these years, then the possibility of continuing to stammer must indeed be a frightening prospect. It seems to us that it is important that we do not collude with this view. We need to help the young person accept the likelihood that they may always stammer to some degree. To do this without taking away their hope and motivation for therapy is indeed a difficult task. Our role is perhaps rather to help young people look at other alternatives; for example, at continuing to stammer but in a less severe way and without allowing the stammer to define the sort of people they are.

Shapiro (1999), however, has warned against making a diagnosis of 'chronic perseverative stuttering syndrome' to the client too early, and especially at the end of a diagnostic interview as described by Cooper (1993). Shapiro described prognosis as 'a dynamic, rather than static entity ... one's prognosis fluctuates with different factors'. We remember making this kind of mistake with a mature teenager, telling him at the end of his first session, in what we thought was a gentle, sensitive way, that there was no cure for stammering. We still can see his face, tears and a look of utter dejection. We have learned, we hope from this experience, to temper the truth with an empathic understanding of the person's individual situation.

Working with Parents

We would adhere to the view held by Rustin *et al* (1991, p89) that 'the adolescent is still part of a family unit and the clinician must be prepared to learn about and understand the family systems in order to involve the parents in a practical, logical and agreed way'. Rustin *et al* (1995, p69) pointed to the benefits of working with parents, namely:

◆ Maintenance of specific skills taught to the child

◆ Greater parental awareness and understanding of the client's problem

◆ Understanding of the difficulties encountered before, during and after therapy.

Yovetich *et al* (2000, p150) echoed the views of many clinicians in saying, 'any clinician working with CWS [children who stutter] who does not include parents as part of the assessment and therapeutic process may well be undermining their own efforts to help the child'. However, there may be some dilemmas for us in working with parents of this age group. If young people come to trust us, they may tell us things that they have been unable or unwilling to discuss with their parents. If we meet with parents separately from their children, the children may be concerned that we will breach their confidence. However, if we only meet parents in the company of their child, parents may feel constrained about expressing some of their underlying concerns or in giving us information that they do not want to share with their child. While we wish to encourage open and honest communication in families, we also recognise the rights of individuals to express their feelings and share information in the knowledge that what they say will remain confidential.

We have no easy answers to this dilemma, and can only suggest that the approach we take will vary from family to family. We wish to avoid, at all costs, a feeling in either young people or their parents that we are talking behind their backs, and we would certainly see it in the best interests of all concerned to open channels of communication between family members wherever possible. Negotiation seems to us to be the key.

Williams (1987) wrote a useful chapter for teenagers who stammer. It outlines specific difficulties which young people and their parents can have about stammering, such as: 'Do your parents act like stuttering is something they don't want to talk about?'; 'Do your parents think that if you really tried you could stop your stuttering?'. Asking young people and their parents to read the chapter between sessions can facilitate talking about things that had not previously been discussed openly. This material can be followed up in discussion in the clinic.

Markham (1990) looked at how adults may identify signs of stress in children, and at some of the possible causal factors. She gives examples of how parents can be helped to 'stress-proof' their children, through improved nutrition, ensuring adequate sleep, use of relaxation techniques and 'positive thinking' and, most importantly of all, by fostering a home environment in which open communication is encouraged. The book covers all ages and stages of childhood, and contains useful ideas which may be applied to any of the stages of stammering and to wider issues such as divorce, bereavement and abuse.

CONCLUSION

Van Riper wrote of his own very negative feelings in his teenage years as a person who stammers, in a publication intended for this age group:

> 'But the worst part of them was that I felt not only helpless but hopeless. How was I ever to get a job or to be able to support myself? How was I ever to get married and raise a family? I felt naked in a world full of steel knives. I thought of suicide and tried it once but failed at that too.' (1987, p72)

Van Riper went on to describe his success in later life, both personally (marriage and children) and professionally (including giving speeches, appearing on television and making films). He initially leaves his young reader to assume that he has been cured, but goes on to confess that he has continued to stammer all his life. He explains that his way of coping with his stammer was not by hiding from, avoiding or fighting stammering, but rather through acceptance and learning to stammer more easily. He points to the many others he has known whose lives have been equally fulfilling despite their stammers, because of the positive attitudes they have developed.

Publications such as these can be helpful in promoting discussion about the future, and in aiding young people and their parents to look at options. By using behaviours that aim to hide or avoid stammering, young people are more likely to limit their choices and narrow their horizons. By being open and confronting the stammer, they may be helped to anticipate an adulthood that can include stammering, but still allow them to develop their potential.

The use of group therapy programmes is well established in the field of fluency disorders. In the first edition of *Working with Dysfluent Children* (Stewart & Turnbull, 1995), we wrote that group programmes were less well established for children than for adults. Things have changed greatly since then, and groups are now seen as an important, if not essential, therapy option. This development may be a response to the increasing demand for efficient use of therapy time and resources, but it is to be hoped that it is also a development which has arisen out of proven positive outcomes. Certainly, our use of group therapy programmes would suggest it has major benefits for the children and is a positive experience for clinicians.

ADVANTAGES

Reduced Feelings of Isolation

A group approach can reduce an individual's anxiety by helping him realise he is not alone in having the feelings and experiences associated with non-fluency. It can also give the individual an awareness of the variety of non-fluency by observing its different forms and manifestations in others. In addition, group therapy usually means that a number of clinicians meet together to manage the group and, thus, professional isolation can be reduced.

Increased Feelings of Support

By mixing with other children, group members may come to feel that the group is a safe haven where they can express their fears and anxieties, as well as their joys and successes. That sense of support may remain after the group has ended, and we are aware of friendships which have been maintained long after a group programme has finished. Clinicians, too, can feel supported by their colleagues in the regime. Students or less experienced clinicians can use the group as a learning experience and gradually increase their confidence, through first observing, then leading small groups, perhaps as a way into striking off on their own.

Improved Clinical Management

We have found that group therapy is a regime which can enable clinicians to deal more effectively with non-fluency in some children. We have experience of children for whom the group represented a turning point in therapy, and sometimes in their approach to life in general. Individual therapy may be a cosy situation that is non-threatening and equally non-challenging for an individual; a group may place him in a more challenging environment and, therefore, change can result.

Non-participation or reluctance to speak can be quite difficult to handle in individual therapy; however, in a group, peers can put children under much more pressure than the individual clinician and they can feel excluded and isolated in a way that is difficult to emulate in individual therapy. There are other children among whom group interactions can precipitate behaviour which has not been observed in a one-to-one situation. A child who appears endearing in one-to-one therapy can be found to be manipulating in a group therapy. Thus, group therapy may be a more realistic setting in which children can experiment and experience change.

In addition, the types of activities that can be used in a group setting can be more varied and diverse than those used in one-to-one therapy. Monitoring and feedback become the responsibility of the whole group, and not just the remit of the clinician. In some instances a child might value the opinion of their peers more than that of a professional, and this can be used to great effect in a group programme.

Finally, at a time when the profession has to account for time and resources, group therapy may be seen as an efficient method of treatment by those needing to attract service contracts.

DISADVANTAGES

Lack of Experience

There is no doubt that facilitating or leading a group can be very daunting. In fact, even after years of experience, we both continue to feel apprehensive at the start of a new group. Now we realise that to feel nervous in this situation is human, but for those clinicians embarking on their first group it is difficult to grasp this perspective.

We recommend that, where possible, inexperienced clinicians go and visit other groups and get involved in their management. Even if the groups visited are substantially different from those that are planned, a clinician can learn a lot about group dynamics and facilitation in a linear way. If a regular commitment to visit another group is not possible, then another option would be a cross-sectional approach, that is, a series of 'one off' visits to different group programmes. In this instance, a clinician would be unable to follow group processes and see the changing roles and perspectives that groups develop over time; she would, however, be able to observe contrasting styles and approaches, which could help in her own decision making.

Less Attention for the Individual

There may be some children for whom group therapy is inappropriate because they are unable to share attention. Their need for individual attention may be such that they cannot share or participate in activities outside an individual relationship or they may have specific problems which need to be addressed separately (such as parental disharmony) and, as a result, would disrupt group dynamics.

Changing Construing

Membership of a group, by definition, means the sharing of a common goal and can mean sharing a common feature, behaviour and/or characteristic. We have already discussed the fine line we tread between the three categories of stammering. It may be that a child erroneously placed in a group may be moved into reconstruing of his difficulties; perhaps a child with early stammering placed with those with borderline stammers may become more aware of the non-fluencies in his own speech and attempt to struggle through them in ways similar to other group members. We must consider carefully our selection of clients for group therapy, and this will be discussed in more detail further on in this chapter.

Practical Difficulties

There are a number of practical considerations which make group therapy a difficult option.

Suitable accommodation

Space within many community and hospital settings is at a premium, and rooms that can accommodate several children, parents and perhaps teachers at the appropriate time can be difficult to find.

Lack of support

This may also pose a problem. Clinicians may find it impossible to enrol the help of a co-worker, even an assistant or volunteer; in such a situation, in our opinion, it would be very difficult and exhausting to run a group single-handedly. Clinicians may struggle to get the support of parents and schools; parents may be unable or unwilling to bring children, or schools may not wish to be involved or give the children the necessary time away from class work.

Working conditions

For some clinicians, these may also cause difficulties. The type and size of some districts or trusts can restrict therapy choices. Case loads may make group therapy an impossible option; client numbers may be too small or prevent the formation of a homogeneous group, and levels of attendance in certain areas may be too erratic for group cohesion.

Follow-up

Group therapy cannot and should not be an end in itself. Group therapy may take children part way through a process or uncover issues that need further exploration. In the absence of suitable follow-up options, group therapy may not be viable.

GUIDELINES FOR ORGANISING GROUPS

Before considering programmes for children of different ages and stages of non-fluency, we will outline some basic guidelines based on our own experiences with groups.

Aims

It is important to set clear aims before embarking upon a group programme. Therapeutic objectives and session plans seem to emerge more easily out of aims that have been well defined beforehand. In addition, children, carers and other professionals appear more able to commit themselves when they understand what the purpose of the group is to be. It is worth considering the importance of attitude change in addition to more obvious fluency-enhancing aims and the involvement of others in the process. (This is a point to which we will return in this chapter.)

Group Composition

When thinking about group composition, ideally it is important to strike a balance between groups that are too similar and do not stimulate change in individuals and groups that are too dissimilar and pose too much of a threat to the individual child.

This is all very well when there is a choice to be made, but often clinicians are not in a position in which they have a pool of clients from whom to choose. Caseloads are not always as homogeneous or as heterogeneous as we would wish. Like Benson (1987), we have found that a narrow age band works best, as it is easier to manage similar interests and abilities. The exception to this would be an older child who is at a younger level in terms of his social and emotional development. Benson also has some useful pointers regarding the sex mix in children's groups. She favours mixed-sex groups as a general rule, but in her experience 5–7-year-olds and 14–17-year-olds manage these relationships best. In contrast 8–13-year-olds tend to split into single-sex subgroups, which can make group cohesion difficult.

Size

The 'right' size for a group depends on a number of factors: the age of the children, accommodation, the number of clinicians available to lend a hand, the experience of the clinicians, and the type of group. For example, a pre-school group with little support is likely to be kept to a small number of clients, perhaps three. However, an adolescent group in whom social interaction is paramount will probably have larger numbers.

There are some basic principles we should be aware of when considering the size of a group. With smaller numbers, we can develop an intimate atmosphere and maximise support and opportunities to participate, and there is likely to be more consensus in the group. With larger groups, there may be an increase in the number of personal relationships in the group, an opportunity to tackle more complex problems, and use the creativity that a larger group generates, but this may be at the expense of the formation of sub-groups, the time taken to problem solve, and the need for greater management.

Meetings

Frequency and duration of each group session, and length of the group programme, are again dependent on other issues (aim of group, client, support available, accommodation and so on). We have tended to favour groups meeting once per week for a relatively short duration, perhaps up to one hour, for pre-school children (and their parents) and school-aged children, and longer meetings for adolescents; we then use intensive programmes to achieve more short-term aims. (Specifically with regard to intensive groups for school-aged children, we have experimented with several different times during a year. To date, the best attended and best supported by teachers and parents seems to be the week before the final week of the summer term.)

Finally, with regard to the length of group therapy programmes, Benson (1987) made a valuable point that the greater the risks to be tackled by the individual child, the greater the need for time to be taken in the group to build up trust, cohesion and safety.

Attendance

At the beginning of each group programme, we stress the importance of full attendance, noting that absences are only permitted in the event of earthquake, nuclear attack or plague (and even in these circumstances a note from home would be required)! We provide telephone contact numbers for each family, so that we can be contacted should a child be unable to attend any session.

Generally, once the group has started we would not introduce new members, as we feel this does affect the forming process of the group. However, situations have arisen in which we have not followed our own guidelines; for example, children have been referred and/or assessed late, but otherwise would have attended from the beginning. In such circumstances we would consider whether it would disrupt the group significantly, and whether the child himself could cope with entering an established group. We may adapt some group activities when a new child is introduced, returning to some 'getting to know you' type of games to allow him to become familiar with the group members and they with him. We would not introduce several new members at one time into a new group without some radical restructuring of the programme, and new members would not be introduced once the group has become established.

If a child fails to attend over several sessions, we make every effort to contact him and ask him to attend, or come and talk to the clinicians on an individual basis to discuss his attendance problems. If there are genuine difficulties, we try to keep the child in touch with group activities by sending handouts to his home and recounting events on the telephone where possible. When a child continues to miss sessions without explanation, he is sent a letter withdrawing him from the programme and asking him/his parents to contact us should therapy be required in the future.

Accommodation

The importance of the right sort of venue was brought home to us when we had singular problems with one or two group meetings involving adult clients. In the wrong sort of setting, group interaction and cohesion can be affected, apart from the fact that clients feel physically uncomfortable, restricted and de-motivated.

Ideally, the venue should match the aims of the group, with space for small-group work, access to other areas (for example a coffee/tea bar) when social interaction is an issue, and a general atmosphere that is appropriate to achieve the objectives which are targeted. In reality, very often we make do with what is available or what we can get.

Planning

It is our belief that adequate planning can be the issue upon which the success of a group may depend. For that reason, we schedule planning meetings with all clinicians (and helpers, whenever possible) some time before the first session.

Our first meeting is usually concerned with setting aims and objectives for the group: what do we want to achieve, what do we want the children to be able to do/feel at the end of the programme? Once that is established, we look at more practical considerations, such as dates, times, finding an appropriate venue and so on. We might also discuss clients suitable for the group at this stage, including referrals that we have received from other clinicians, and a list is usually drawn up by one of the team. In subsequent planning meetings, our main focus is designing the content of the programme.

It is interesting to note at this point that we do not tend to use commercially available programmes in their entirety, nor do we use the same programme twice. Some people may regard this as folly, and certainly we cannot be criticised for taking an easy option! On reflection, we think it is our personal preference; we are more comfortable designing our own material and it does ensure that the content accurately reflects our thoughts and our aims, and matches the current needs of our clients. In addition, when we have returned to material we have used previously, like many other clinicians, we can be very self-critical and realise that we have moved on in our own thinking and beliefs about what we regard as appropriate. Thus we hope our therapy is dynamic and reflects the changing face of what we know and do not know about stammering.

Benson (1987, p37) discussed some common mistakes made in planning. Included in the list were:

- Failures to link the programme and group objectives
- Programme is too rigid because of over-planning and failure to allow for spontaneous and unexpected incidents and events
- Programme is too little/too much task-centred
- Programme is too little/too much person-centred
- Activity becomes an end rather than a means
- Failure to review or evaluate as a way of fine-tuning or redesigning the programme.

We would like to make a number of suggestions regarding planning groups. These are based on our experiences and therefore may not be generally applicable. We include them here only as ideas to consider.

Type of group

First of all, it is necessary to think about what type of group would be most appropriate to meet the aims and the needs of the clients. We have several options open to us: residential/non-residential, intensive/non-intensive, parents-only/teachers-only groups, and groups in which others (such as siblings or peers) take an active part. There are advantages and disadvantages to each particular type of group. For example, intensive groups are useful for the establishment of new behaviours or techniques, whereas non-intensive programmes can allow us to build on children's experiences in a more gradual way. We will discuss the appropriateness of different types of programmes for different types of children later in this next section.

Planning content

When designing the content of a programme, we have found it useful to break down the process into stages. These stages may relate to specific objectives or may, in the case of week-long intensive programmes, relate to time (a session, a day). For example, as we will discuss later, one programme took the theme of 'Me as I want to be'; we subdivided this into a number of key areas such as, 'Me as I want to be at home', 'Me as I want to be at school'. As it was a week's programme, we then assigned an individual area to a day and designed activities specific to that area for each day.

It is important to make sure that a variety of activities is planned for each session. As a general guideline, we start and end a session/day with activities that draw the group together; a sharing or review around a particular theme or a game that may start or end with a positive experience. For the remainder of the session, we blend activities that require large-group participation, small-group work, and work carried out in pairs and individually.

In the early stages of a group, we carry out one or more activities variously known as 'meshing/gelling/ice-breaking/trust-building' activities. With little ones, it may also be necessary to include a settling time and, if their parents are leaving for their own group, some space should be made for them to move away at a comfortable point. We also may do less work in the large group in the early stages of the group's development. In some instances, we may choose to talk for children, to ease them into the rather daunting situation of talking in front of a big group of unfamiliar peers (for example, introduce them to the group, including saying their name). We generally include an activity in which some ground rules are negotiated and laid down by the group, clinicians, students and helpers together at an early stage. These 'rules' can range from the very practical (such as who is bringing the chocolate biscuits or how would individuals like the group to respond when they get stuck) to rules about conduct and personal space.

How much is planned before the group begins?

In our pre-group planning sessions, one of our team of clinicians acts as scribe and takes responsibility for the recording and subsequent typing and copying of the plans. Included in each session plan is an estimated start and finish time for each activity and the equipment needed. At the time of planning, decisions are made as to which clinician is taking responsibility for supplying visual aids, equipment and so on. Responsibilities are shared out between the team, to ensure that no one clinician has too much of a burden to shoulder in addition to her other casework. However, other than assigning a technical role (for example, camera person for video recording), we do not usually decide at this stage which clinician will direct, lead or facilitate which parts of the session. Such decisions seem to be made quite naturally at the time. It may be that we have worked together in groups with other clinicians sufficiently to know what strengths and skills we have at our disposal. It is important to play off those strengths, and we would seek not to place less experienced colleagues and students in situations in which they did not feel comfortable or prepared. Thus some negotiation of their role in leading areas of a programme may be discussed at the beginning or at the end of a session in preparation for the next day. (Further suggestions regarding the valuable roles that students can play will be made later in this section.)

We make sure that the administrative chores are carried out alongside the planning. One of our team is a fastidious letter writer, and all planning stops while the appropriate letter is composed. This is a useful discipline and one that ensures important planning points are not overlooked (such as does the caretaker/security officer know we will be in the department after locking up time?).

No matter how efficient and well-prepared a group has been, in our experience it is necessary to return to the plans immediately before the commencement of the group. Either as a group of clinicians or as individuals, it is necessary to double-check that rooms have been booked, officials are aware of our imminent arrival, items of equipment have been purchased and have arrived (at the right place), and that the descriptions of the planned activities make sense some weeks after their inception.

Finally, in cases where attendance has been poor in the past, we may also remind some children and their parents that the group is going ahead.

Pre-Group Meeting

We have found it useful, before some of our group therapy programmes, to hold a short introductory session for all participants – clinicians, children and their parents. This would take place usually a few days or the week before the beginning of the group and would be in the same venue, to allow participants to become familiar with the route from home, the parking problems and the accommodation itself. The aims of such a meeting are:

◆ To allow everyone to get to know each other a little before the programme starts

◆ To present the programme to the participants and parents in a non-threatening manner

◆ To convey some practical details about the running of the programme and any essential/non-negotiable rules (such as leaving the premises without consent).

A TYPICAL PROGRAMME

The Pre-Group Meeting

A typical outline for an evening pre-group meeting might take the following form:

19:00   Arrival of children and parents.

Clinicians and helpers provide refreshments and talk informally to group members on an individual basis.

19:20   Formal presentation by one or two clinicians, which would include the following information:

(i)   Introduction of team to group and introduction of group members to group (carried out by the clinicians).

(ii)   Background to the group; how and why it came about.

(iii)   Purpose, goals and objectives of the group.

(iv)   Content of the programme, day-to-day or session-by-session outlines, including timing, venues and duration of the sessions.

(v)   Items to be provided by team, equipment, finances and so on to be provided by group members/carers.

(vi)   Evaluation and feedback, including details to be provided at the end of the programme (such as a final report, an individual interview).

(vii)	Consent forms for video/audio recording, administration of first aid, parental consent for older children to leave the premises unaccompanied, and so on.
(viii)	Possible problems; what to do in the event of illness, provision for the unexpected cancellation of a session/sessions, accidents, misconduct.

19:45   Simple trust-building exercise (see Brandes & Phillips, 1978; Rustin & Kuhr, 1989).

20:00–20:15   Closing comments by clinician.

We have found these pre-group meetings to be particularly useful in allaying the fears of some more apprehensive children. On occasions, we have lost children before groups have actually started, as the fear and dread associated with a new speaking situation has prevented them from taking even a first step. Being able to make that step with a family member and being reassured that it will be a pleasant, non-threatening experience is often sufficient to allow them to proceed with future attendances.

Roles within a Group

Clinicians

We thoroughly enjoy working with a team of clinicians in a group programme. The roles that we adopt individually in any programme will depend upon the needs of the children, the needs that the programme dictates, and our own strengths and weaknesses.

In our groups, no one clinician takes the lead throughout the entire group; rather, the role of leader rotates around the team and this seems to help the group members relate to clinicians whom they may not have met before in the same way as more familiar team members. This rotation also allows us to use the skills of certain clinicians to the advantage of the programme and enables others to take more of a back seat on occasions, acting as observers of children's behaviour, the activity and/or the group processes in general.

The team of clinicians is usually a mix of experienced and less experienced individuals seeking to develop their skills. Thus there is almost a hidden agenda of clinical training and development taking place alongside the aspects of communication. We recommend a minimum of two experienced clinicians involved with a group of any age at any one time. There are other situations in which a greater number of professionals would be desirable: for example, when taking children out of clinic premises, in activities involving individual feedback, and with smaller children whose physical needs may be less predictable. If larger numbers of qualified staff are not available, then it may be possible to enlist helpers and/or students, at least for some parts of the programme (discussed in the section on the use of students and observers below).

The family

The role of family members in group therapy again depends on factors relating to the nature of the group, age of the children, aims and objectives and so on. Irrespective of these fundamental issues, it is crucial to the success of the programme that the children are supported at home, whether they are learning new skills or attempting to change their own feelings and attitudes to speech. We depend on parents especially to help us reach our objectives, but siblings too may have a part to play. With little ones, very often parents need to be around to settle the children and provide a sense of security in an unfamiliar setting. We would encourage parents to move away from the group at a point when the child appears happy; this may mean taking a back seat in the same room, or moving to an adjacent room (ideally with observational facilities into the children's room). This helps the children to establish their own place within a group, develop relationships and not use the parents to opt out at critical times when life gets a bit tough for them in the group.

When we have been able to separate children and parents, it has been useful to use this time for them to meet as a group themselves. Interesting issues about the child at home, interactions with other family members, difficulties in handling non-fluency, and useful learning points can all be discussed, to the benefit of parents and clinicians.

In the case of older children, the situation is often a little different: children and parents may be happy to separate – and, indeed, often prefer it! With groups of this age range, we have involved parents in a variety of ways:

◆ To motivate children
◆ To provide background information about their child pertinent to the group programme
◆ To observe their children in a certain activity or situation and provide feedback to them
◆ To practise skills outside the group
◆ To provide specific input in sessions relating to interactions in the home/ involving siblings
◆ To provide specific input in sessions relating to social skills/ assertiveness/negotiation
◆ To help in problem-solving particular difficulties for individuals.

One note of caution regarding parental involvement in group therapy: we have had instances when asking parents to contribute in activities involving the whole group, such as group discussions, has highlighted specific problems that the adults have in these situations. We need to be mindful that children may not be alone in finding these circumstances anxiety-provoking.

Teachers

Because of the pressure which teachers are under, generally we have found it difficult to involve teachers on an intensive basis in group programmes. We have, however, had excellent support from schools and much encouragement for our work. Teachers have observed group therapy programmes, both intensive and non-intensive, and have made some valuable comments and observations.

With regard to intensive programmes, in recent years we have devoted one session to the child in school. Teachers have been released to attend these sessions and activities have included:

◆ Clinician providing information on the nature of stammering

◆ Teachers and children working together to solve individual difficulties in the class

◆ Teachers discussing their perspective on the non-fluency.

When a child's pattern of dysfluency is characterised by more covert symptoms, it is useful to have the child and the teacher talk together informally about the child's feelings in certain speaking situations. The clinician may act as a facilitator for the child, helping him realise that his problem is not construed by the outside world (in this case the classroom teacher) in the same way as he construes it. Similarly, the teacher may come to reconstrue the lack of overt symptoms as masking an issue of real concern to the child.

In groups that take place at the end of the summer term, we often request the attendance of two teachers for one child. Where the child is moving schools (from junior to a secondary/high school, for example) we would ask a teacher from the new school, preferably the form tutor, to attend in addition to the current class teacher. This has proved a useful exchange of information and, with a teacher on his side, the child is helped to see the new school situation as less threatening.

Use of students/observers

We have found speech and language therapy students to be invaluable in running group programmes, so much so that now we request that students are placed with us. In addition, we do have occasional visiting clinicians – individuals who are interested in finding out about groups, different therapy options, different client groups and so on.

How we utilise the developing skills of students or observer depends on a number of factors, including the nature of the group therapy programme, the abilities and level of confidence of the visitor and the children or adolescents themselves. As a minimal requirement, we expect all visitors to take on basic responsibilities:

◆ To assist in planning and administrative tasks wherever possible

◆ To help with general management of the groups (such as room preparation, gathering and maintaining equipment)

◆ To observe group processes and individual clients

◆ To monitor and evaluate in line with group targets

◆ To assist in report writing and the debriefing sessions as appropriate.

Over and above these basic requirements, we are keen for observers to use the experience in a way that is useful for them in terms of their particular level of development and individual needs. One way of structuring their involvement is to create levels or a hierarchy of activities which are increasingly demanding and through which students could choose to progress, or attempt to gain experience at each level. An example of such a hierarchy would be:

1   Working with individual group members on tasks assigned in the group

2   Working with pairs of children on tasks assigned in the group

3   Working alongside small groups of children on particular tasks, and/or facilitating activities (such as discussions, role plays) carried out in small groups

4   Leading the whole group in an activity, including presenting the activity, explaining the task, organising the group or smaller units of the group to carry out the task, gathering and sharing the results, and summing up

5   Leading a session. This would involve briefing other members of the team on the content and timing of the activities, delegating where appropriate, and coordinating or leading several activities as in 4.

Such a structure is based on group activities. There are, however, other approaches that we have used which relate more to the children and their needs. Lees & Boyle (1993), for example, suggested assigning one student to one client per session. The student then acts as a mentor for that particular child, assisting him in any way appropriate (such as providing feedback on a particular skill being acquired, helping in a problem-solving approach) throughout the allotted time. At the end of the session/day, the student then has the responsibility to feed back to the remainder of the team her client's progress, any problems, successes, and areas to be noted for the next session. For that next session the student is assigned a different group member, and thus students and group members rotate for the duration of the group programme.

A modification of this approach is to assign a child to a particular student for the total length of the group programme. Thus the student would work with the child individually, work alongside any pairs and small groups into which he was placed, but also participate as a general group/team member in any large group activities. It is important for the student to balance her mentor role with her role in the group as a whole and be aware of not shadowing the child so closely that spontaneous interaction with other group members is inhibited. We have found that this method works particularly well with children identified as having needs that are difficult to manage in a group situation; children with literacy problems, difficulties in understanding, behavioural difficulties and those with general social and emotional immaturities can be helped considerably to cope, given this arrangement. It can also prove advantageous when a student is required to gather information on one client, for example, for analysis purposes or in order to write a detailed case report.

Recording

We use different types of recording to fulfil a number of purposes in our group programmes. First, DVD/video and audio recording and playback are often used in a number of interactive activities. For example, adolescents may carry dictaphones when carrying out a survey on a given topic outside the clinic/hospital premises. Younger children have used video equipment to record their own news broadcast or advertisements. In these instances, the use of these facilities can add a further dimension to the activity: a fairly low-key situation may be given the additional pressure of a 'performance', and the presence of the equipment may create a more real situation for the children. In terms of the playback of the recording, children usually enjoy reliving their performance.

Once in a while there are individuals who do not react well to hearing and seeing themselves as others do. One of the authors remembers well, as a toddler, having a meal with friends of the family, during which the proceedings were covertly audiotaped. When the tape was replayed, everyone laughed at the conversation and silly comments that had been made during the meal, but for the toddler it felt as though the laughter was directed at her and her immature-sounding voice. It was not a game for her, but became an intrusive and undermining experience.

We must take care that individuals are given constructive, balanced feedback. Comments on behaviours that require active change or modification should be counterbalanced by positive observations to reinforce and consolidate good behaviours. The use of checklists can be helpful here, as they ensure that feedback is specific and to the point. Everyone should have an opportunity to comment and receive the views of others; there is nothing worse than no one saying anything at all about a particular child's efforts. We have also used DVD/video- and audio-taping in a more routine way, as a way of making a record of individual and group progress and evaluating therapy. When note-keeping may seem more intrusive and disrupts the flow of interactions, the DVD or video recorder placed in the corner can quietly record events and becomes, after a while, part of the furniture. Playback can focus on different aspects of the group dynamics, and may provide a valuable learning experience for students wishing to obtain objective feedback on aspects of their own skills.

In whatever way DVD/video or audio recorders are used, it is important to obtain the consent of the children and their parents before their use. We have a standard consent form that we use in Leeds which, once signed, allows us to use the recordings for a specified time period, for clinical and limited teaching and research purposes.

We have also found it essential that at least one member of our therapy team should be familiar with the equipment and have a basic knowledge of common problems and their remedies (or know a technician who does). Time must be allowed for this clinician to set up and test the equipment before the exercise. We have learned from painful experience about tapes that have not recorded, or recordings that have no sound, and so in this area, especially, we try to be well prepared.

In the absence of DVD or video facilities and for some special tasks, pen and paper may be a good substitute. Recently, we have used a 'diary monitoring' book. This book is used by every member of the team to record particular behaviours, feelings, and observations about individual children. It is kept in a central, secure place and can be filled in at any time of the day/session, by any clinician or helper. Indeed, it is part of our individual responsibilities to try and record some observations on each child at some point during the session. This record has proved invaluable when, at some later stage, we try to evaluate an individual child's progress and the outcomes of the programme in general terms.

Debriefing

At the end of each session, the team of clinicians and helpers meets to discuss what has happened, record significant events and review the plans for the next session, replanning where necessary.

In addition, at the end of each group therapy programme a debriefing meeting is held. This meeting, which usually takes place the week after the end of the course, is attended by all clinicians and helpers. (Generally, the students have come to the end of their placement and therefore cannot attend; their debriefing and feedback on clinical skills and so on takes place separately.) The debriefing takes the form of a general evaluation of the programme: whether the aims were achieved, which activities were particularly useful or particularly unproductive, how the programme could be improved. As a result of this discussion, a summary of the group and its outcomes is written by the team and key learning points are written down for use when the next programme is planned.

The clinicians then divide into pairs and write reports on the individual children. The group summary forms the first portion of the report and, therefore, the clinicians need only consider progress and outcomes relating to particular children. It is at this stage that the 'diary' proves invaluable. Points made in the book serve to jog memories and we find it much easier to write the reports, quoting specific instances and examples of behaviour as a result.

Some time later, a debriefing session is arranged for the children and their parents. During the session, further discussion of the group programme is carried out and there is an opportunity for us to hear the views of the consumers. We also use this session to feed back our observations and feelings to the children and their parents. Some time is set aside for individual clinicians to meet and discuss in private the reports on the children. Both the parents and children are present, and are encouraged to voice their opinions and comments on our report about them and the group programme in general. This can provide valuable insights and information on what effect therapy has had in situations outside clinic. Finally, what might constitute the next step for the child is considered. Various options might be suggested by the clinician, and these are talked about in clinical and practical terms.

After the Group

We believe that it is important that group therapy programmes are not seen as ends in themselves. They can be powerful initiators in terms of moving and motivating individuals into new areas of change. It is essential that this is then followed up and appropriate provision made to support the children in a continuing way, should this be required. Options that may be considered are as follows:

◆ Discharge (with referral to self-help group, other support agency such as the British Stammering Association (BSA) or other agency).

◆ Infrequent support
  – Periodic review in clinic, school or at home
  – Individual and/or parental counselling
  – Attendance at monthly follow-up group meetings
  – Attendance at future intensive groups during school holidays.

◆ Regular support
  – Non-intensive
  – Individual therapy
  – Group therapy
  – Intensive
  – Individual therapy
  – Group therapy

◆ Individual counselling of child and/or parents.

These options or range of alternatives may be made available in a department or district. In the absence of facilities, clinicians may consider referring the child to another district, with the consent of the child, carer and purchaser of care.

Having Fun

Our final message about groups is positive: we continue to find them stimulating, challenging and satisfying. We enjoy watching children change, develop, maximise existing skills and discover new ones. Groups can be hard work and often wear us out. We need to share what can often be a heavy load with our colleagues and benefit from their help and support. Above all, we like groups!

THE GROUP AS A WHOLE

In any group programme, for whatever stage of non-fluency, we must have our eyes focused on the group as a whole. We have found it all too easy to fall into the trap of carrying out individual therapy in groups, that is, spending time on each individual in turn, rather than letting the group function as an entity in its own right. We need to ensure that individual needs are not overlooked, but never to lose sight of the collective effect of the group. Whitaker & Lieberman (1964, p3) pointed out that group processes may affect each person differently and 'the manner in which each patient contributes to, participates in and is affected by the group processes determines to a considerable degree whether he will profit from his group therapy experience, be untouched by it or be alarmed by it'.

THE INDIVIDUAL IN THE GROUP

The groups we will use in this chapter to illustrate our programmes have been organised according to the development of the children's construing of their dysfluency (for example, groups for borderline stammering) or the child's developmental stage (for example, pre-schoolers/reception age-children), or sometimes both (teenage and confirmed stammering). We are aware that it can sometimes be counterproductive to keep together children at the same developmental stage, if their ages and their social development are disparate. A confirmed 9-year-old stammerer is unlikely, for example, to benefit from being in a group of 15-year-olds, but may be far more comfortable in a borderline stammering group with those nearer his own age. Children must be assessed and considered for inclusion in a group on the basis of their own individual factors. Ideally, the group should fit the children, not require them to change in order to meet group criteria. However, we recognise that this may be easier to organise in a district with larger numbers of referrals.

GROUPS FOR PARENTS OF YOUNGER DYSFLUENT CHILDREN

We have already stated that we feel it is most appropriate to intervene with the families of younger dysfluent children, rather than directly with the children. Although we may initially do this on an individual basis, we feel that meeting in a group can also offer some additional advantages in terms of reducing isolation and encouraging discussion.

Aims

1 To create a comfortable atmosphere in which parents feel relaxed and able to express their feelings about their child and dysfluency in an open and honest way.

2 To give parents the opportunity to see how others react to their child's dysfluency, and to help them to explore similarities and differences in their attitudes.

3 To provide some education into the nature of stammering and its development.

4 To consider the approaches which seem to be most helpful to dysfluent children.

5 To help the parents empathise with their children's perception of 'the problem'.

Meetings

It is felt that meetings should take place in the evening in order to make attendance easier. We recognise that there could be problems with arranging child care, and therefore propose only two meetings. Holding these between 19:00 and 21:00, on the same weekday, with two weeks between sessions, seems to suit the majority.

Group Composition

Number of parents

If there are two parents involved in a child's care, admission to the group is generally contingent on the attendance of both. However, if one parent has a genuine reason for not being able to attend (such as working away, shift worker unable to take holiday), we may be prepared to accept the attendance of only one parent. If only one parent is involved in child care, we would try, if possible, to ensure that they are in a group where they are not the only such parent. A group of between 8 and 10 parents is deemed to be small enough for people to feel able to contribute to discussions, but large enough to generate a variety of ideas.

Suitability for group

We feel that, as well as being prepared to attend both sessions, parents should be willing and able to participate in group discussions. In practice this means they may not be invited if their commitment is low or if they feel too uncomfortable to join in discussions. If their English is not at a sufficient level to allow them to participate, we need to endeavour to find suitably trained interpreters. Interpreting in a group situation is a skilled activity if it is not to disrupt the flow of the group.

Children's dysfluency

The group described below is concerned with either pre-schoolers or children in a reception class. Levels of overt dysfluency may vary, and the children may be at either the early or the borderline stages of development.

Previous therapy

In our groups, at least one parent of every child has already been seen for a minimum of one individual session. We feel that, in this way, we can get to know the parents and their individual needs and also ascertain their appropriateness for such a group. All should be concerned to find out more about stammering and to explore new ways of dealing with it.

A TYPICAL PROGRAMME

First Evening

19:00   The clinicians introduce themselves. A brief outline of the two sessions is given.

19:10   Group gelling. We feel that, unless parents are given some time to get to know each other, sufficient trust is not built up for them to feel able to express their feelings in a group of strangers. However, we are also aware that such activities cannot take too long if there is only a total of 4 hours at our disposal. It is therefore useful to use activities that allow people some freedom in what they say, give them a chance to get to know each other, but also feel relevant to the participants' reasons for attending. We are aware from our own experience of attending short courses how introductions can sometimes seem to take an inordinate amount of time, especially if the information gained from them does not seem to be used in any way in the ensuing session.

One way of 'breaking the ice' is to for parents to talk informally about their own families in pairs or small groups. No instructions are given as to content or as to whether dysfluency should be mentioned. Information can be *briefly* fed back to the large group. It is interesting to note what things have been talked about and what is missing; for example, whether the dysfluency features, whether the family picture is particularly rosy or gloomy and so on.

19:40 Handout 3, entitled 'Statements about stammering: true or false?' is given out (p190). In two groups, parents are invited to discuss and reach a consensus as to which of the statements are true and which are false. In the large group, answers are compared with further discussion and therapist input and clarification of any misconceptions. The statements refer both to 'facts', for example, 'More boys than girls stammer' and to attitudes, for example, 'It is important not to discipline children who stammer as much as other children'.

> **Handout: Statements about stammering – true or false?**
> Children who stammer have something wrong with their mouths
> Children who stammer all have brown hair and blue eyes
> Children who stammer are nervous and shy
> Stammering often runs in families
> Children who stammer may get teased
> You should not discuss your child's speaking difficulties with them
> Children's speech is normally fluent
> Some famous people stammer

More boys than girls stammer

It is best to tell a child to say a different word if they find a particular word hard to say

Children stammer because they talk too fast

It is important not to discipline children who stammer as much as other children are disciplined.

20:10 Coffee and informal chat.

20:20 The remainder of the evening is given to looking at both the overt and covert nature of stammering using Sheehan's icebergs (1975). The clinicians explain these two features of stammering and their relevance to its development. Examples are given of icebergs of children at the three developmental stages (early, borderline and confirmed). A handout is given to be taken home, and parents are each invited to compile an iceberg of their own child, to be brought to the next meeting.

Second Evening

19:00 Clinicians recap briefly on the first evening, and outline what is to happen in this session.

19:10 Parents are asked to arrange themselves in alphabetical order of their first name. They then pair up with the person next to them (with some adjustments being made if they find themselves next to their own partner). The pairs are given ideas to help them discuss the icebergs which they have compiled on their child, concerning their feelings about the task, what they feel it may have taught them and any differences between their iceberg and that of their child's other parent.

19:25 Feedback to large group.

19:40 Therapists compile two group icebergs in a rather different way than normal. The first looks at parents and children's feelings during a conversation in which children are fluent. Above the line is written anything the child is believed to be experiencing during such conversations. Typical responses are 'lack of frustration', 'pleasure', 'feeling listened to', 'being corrected more for errors of grammar and speech', 'longer conversations'. Below the line are the parents' experiences in such conversations. These

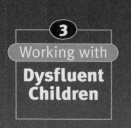
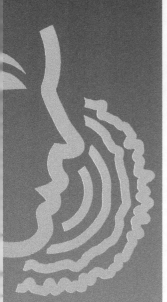

HANDOUT: STATEMENTS ABOUT STAMMERING – TRUE OR FALSE?

Children who stammer have something wrong with their mouths

Children who stammer all have brown hair and blue eyes

Children who stammer are nervous and shy

Stammering often runs in families

Children who stammer may get teased

You should not discuss your child's speaking difficulties with them

Children's speech is normally fluent

Some famous people stammer

More boys than girls stammer

It is best to tell a child to say a different word if they find a particular word hard to say

Children stammer because they talk too fast

It is important not to discipline children who stammer as much as other children are disciplined tend to include such things as 'wanting to prolong talking when it is fluent', 'not needing to make excuses about why you didn't understand' and 'wondering when it is going to get worse again'.

The second iceberg looks in the same way at situations in which children are dysfluent. Parents' perceptions of their children's experiences tend to include awareness of interventions, such as 'speak slowly', having sentences finished for them, being asked for repetitions. Some parents feel that children experience extra patience from them when they are dysfluent, others feel they receive less. Parents' experiences include feelings of frustration, apprehension about the reactions of others and questions about 'Why?'.

Such an exercise brings a raising of perception and a fertile discussion ground. Parents often discover that their own awareness, frustration and anxiety about their child's dysfluencies are far greater than their child's. This process can help them to reconstrue the dysfluency less negatively.

Another factor that can become apparent is that parents often seek causal factors for each specific episode of stammering. Discussions lead to an awareness that very often this is a fruitless exercise, and that stammering does not usually involve such a direct cause-and-effect process.

20:10 Coffee and informal chat.

20:20 The next part of the session is given to looking at ideas to facilitate more natural and pleasurable communication between parents and children, regardless of level of fluency. We feel it is important for clinicians to point out that there is no evidence suggesting that parents are responsible for their children's dysfluency, but that it does seem to be likely that parents can reduce the likelihood of it developing to a further stage and becoming a major issue for children and their families.

Ideas are brainstormed and then discussed. Clinicians offer their own thoughts where appropriate.

20:35 Problem-solving. One of the clinicians offers a hypothetical child-rearing problem (for example, sleep, temper tantrums, fear of new places) and the other leads the group in approaching possible solutions using this technique. The technique is offered as a way of approaching problems that may arise for the children of the parents in the group.

20:55 Closing round. Generally, out of the discussions has come the idea that parents should try to concentrate on and praise children for things other than fluency. We end the evening with a round of 'one thing I will praise my child for'. It is suggested that parents together make a list of a variety of positive aspects of their child and, at home, discuss how they will carry out this praise. Parents may wish to exchange contact details in order to be able to offer each other future support.

GROUPS FOR SCHOOL-AGED BORDERLINE STAMMERING

One of the major benefits of group therapy for this client group is that it can show children that they are not alone, and that stammering occurs in other children with a range of personalities and from a variety of backgrounds. Observing the ways in which these other children approach their dysfluency may open new ways with which the individual can experiment. A vivacious, extrovert 11-year-old in one of our groups, when asked about people he liked and did not like, told the group that he couldn't stand people who were quiet and didn't express their views. This had quite an impact on another extremely shy group member who looked up to this particular boy. Indeed, it appeared to be a trigger to his own participation in the group.

The variety of activities which can be used in group therapy is also an advantage with this group, who can typically become bored quite easily unless material presented is stimulating and catches their imagination. It is useful to vary content and group formation (work in pairs, small groups, large groups, and so on), and to balance sedentary and more active pursuits. In individual therapy, fewer options are available.

Aims

Groups for borderline stammerers may encompass one or more of the following aims:

1   To provide a forum in which dysfluency can be openly discussed, problems aired and solutions discussed.

2   To increase awareness of general communication skills, work on improving them where necessary, and to use self-monitoring as a means of taking pressure off the need to be fluent.

3   To work at a preventative level where appropriate, and to help children understand the dangers of hiding stammering.

4   To increase positive self-worth, regardless of stammering.

5   To provide the children with a means of talking in an easier, more controlled way.

6   To provide a forum for children to practise things that they may have avoided in the past (for example, reading out, asking questions, talking to new people).

7   To help parents understand more about dysfluency, both generally and its individual nature in their own child, to reconstrue it where appropriate and to discover ways in which they can best help their child.

Types of Group

We are aware that it would be possible, but not practicable within the scope of this book, to discuss a variety of different types of group programmes (for example, intensive or non-intensive, teaching social skills or teaching fluency). Instead, we are going to describe just two groups that we have run: one for 6–8-year-olds and the other for children of approximately 8–13 years of age, both within the borderline stammering stage.

Meetings

The groups we will be describing are run on a weekly basis, for one hour a week during the course of one school year. There are no meetings during school holidays. Meetings are held in a city centre NHS location and children attend from all over the city, so may have long journeys. From experience, we find that the most appropriate time for such a group to be held is either first thing in the morning or last thing in the afternoon, to ensure that as little schooling as possible is missed.

Degree of dysfluency

This kind of group is appropriate for children who are aware of and have some concern about their dysfluency. The degree of severity of the overt symptoms is less important. However, if numbers permit, it is best to ensure that children with severe stammers are not placed in groups where they feel very different.

Age of children

We have suggested approximate age ranges, but maturity should also be taken into account. We would, for example, not wish to have a group comprising a mixture of immature 8-year-olds and mature 13-year-olds – a recipe for disaster.

Sex of children

This is an age at which children often form same-sex groupings. We would therefore rarely put a lone girl into a group of boys, unless the child in question felt quite happy with the arrangement. However, in our experience, as long as there are at least two girls, the group usually gels satisfactorily. In fact, we find that the girls are often a calming influence on boys of this age.

Number of clinicians

This will, of course, depend on the size of the group and on how it is organised. We would recommend the involvement of two clinicians wherever possible. Practically, this allows more flexibility (for example, if something urgent crops up or if one of the clinicians is ill). In addition, if parents are involved directly in therapy or if they are merely waiting to collect their child, the availability of more than one therapist provides an opportunity to do some individual counselling as appropriate. It also enables clinicians to discuss any problems with parents as they are occurring.

Involvement of others

Various options are available for the involvement of others:

1   Parents or carers may be invited to attend the sessions. While it may be useful to involve them directly in the group process, both children and parents may well be inhibited by each other's presence. The children may, in addition, not make as close relationships with the other children.

2   Parents or carers may have a regular group of their own. This has a major advantage of allowing parents to express their feelings about the dysfluency, find out how others feel and consider how they can best help their child. However, the organisation of such a group may incur some problems. Both an extra room and an extra clinician are needed. Children whose parents cannot or will not attend are disadvantaged. (We sometimes have children who are brought to the group by volunteers; were this not the case, the children would not be able to receive therapy.)

3   Parents, carers or volunteers can be included for the last part of each session. This can be a useful way of ensuring that home practice tasks are identified and explained. In addition, there may be occasional group sessions arranged for them to attend, sometimes with and sometimes without the children. They can also meet together informally while waiting for their child, and may have the opportunity to talk briefly to the clinician and arrange further appointments where necessary. (It should be noted that, before children are admitted to the groups, they have been assessed and they and/or their parents, where possible, will have been given some individual therapy.) This is the compromise solution that we find most practical in our own working environment.

4   Teachers may be invited to attend one or more of the weekly sessions. We have experimented with this idea but found it to be impracticable, as a one-hour session gives too short a time for anything useful to be achieved. In addition, it has proved almost impossible to organise to enable all teachers to attend. We prefer, therefore, to arrange a separate group, as described in Chapter 10 on schools.

A TYPICAL PROGRAMME FOR 6–8-YEAR-OLDS

For this age range, we recommend that clinicians have a range of interesting stickers to give out readily, in order to keep the children's interest and motivation. Other incentives we use include 'a special seat' for good behaviour, and allowing a particular child to call the parents in at the end of the group.

We would suggest 8 as a good number of participants in this sort of group, and no more than 10, especially if it includes some with a poor attention span.

Session 1

Parents and children have separate groups, so it may be necessary to involve an extra therapist.

Parents' group

◆ Introduction by clinician.

◆ Parents introduce themselves and tell others a little about their children.

◆ Clinician outlines the format of the group (aims are to increase confidence, improve general communication skills, promote ideas for fluency and stop the development of more concerning stammering symptoms).

◆ Clinician mentions that there will be an individual review at the end of the group, when further therapy options will be discussed.

◆ An appropriate video is shown (for example 'Time to talk' produced by the Michael Palin Centre). The aim is to examine helpful and unhelpful parental behaviour.

◆ Discussion of the video and of positive parental behaviours.

◆ Questions.

Children's group

◆ Introductions by clinicians.

◆ Children have a 'bingo sheet' with six squares each containing a picture – a house, an animal, some food, a school, a child, and a family group. Each child has to talk to six children and find out something about them in relation to each picture: What is their house like? Do they have a pet? What is their favourite food? What is the name of their school? A friend's name? The people in their family?

◆ The group meets together and shares what has been learned about each child in turn, under each category.

◆ 'Same and different'. On a flip chart, we do a tally on physical characteristics (for example, number of children with black/brown/blond/curly/straight hair, number of short/tall children, and so on). The aim of this exercise is to show the children that everyone is like others in some ways and different in others.

◆ Other similarities and differences are discussed (hobbies, likes and dislikes), leading on to looking at differences in the way people speak.

◆ Change is discussed. Which of the things we have discussed can we change, and what can't we change? We can change the length of our hair but not the colour of our eyes, for example. We can change our hobbies but not our height. Speech can be included in the discussion – both general aspects and fluency.

◆ Children say one thing they could change and one thing they couldn't. (Children frequently mention their 'bumpy talking', almost always as something they can change.)

◆ Parents come in. A volunteer is chosen to help the clinician explain to the parents what they have been doing – there is always a clamour to do this.

◆ Homework is given. Children draw a picture of themselves and write down things they do and do not like about themselves.

Session 2

◆ Homework is reviewed. Pictures are stuck on the wall and children outline one thing they like and one thing they do not like about themselves.

◆ The clinician tells a story about a child who always did the same thing, day after day – got up at the same time, had the same breakfast, played with the same friends, watched the same television programme, and so on. The children are invited to look at each activity and say what the child could have experimented with changing, for example, tried Weetabix instead of cornflakes, got up 10 minutes earlier/later.

◆ Children each decide on a change they would like to try out during the week.

◆ Identification exercise – bumpy speech. Clinicians demonstrate and children practise different ways of being bumpy (fast rate, choppy, hard attack, repetitions, and so on) while they guess what picture is on a card which the clinician describes. This leads to a discussion about the 'best' type of bumpy talking, that is, one with less force and tension.

◆ Parents come in. A volunteer helps explain the session.

◆ Homework is given. Children identify what they like and dislike about their talking, and both parents and children experiment with changing some aspect of their normal daily routine. At home, they discuss how easy or difficult this was to do.

Session 3

◆ Homework is reviewed. Children each say one thing they like and one thing they do not like about their speech.

◆ Brainstorm 'when people's speech is bumpy'. A tally is taken, and put on a flip chart, of all the different situations mentioned and the numbers of children finding each situation difficult.

◆ Clinicians have a conversation using both easy and bumpy talking. Children take turns to give the clinician a token when they hear easy talking. They can take the token away if they identify a bumpy word. The children have to demonstrate how to say a word in an easy way when the clinician has bumped on it.

◆ Parents come in. A volunteer explains the session.

◆ Homework is given. Children demonstrate bumpy and smooth talking in single words to their parents, while naming pictures or objects.

Session 4

◆ Homework is reviewed. Children tell us how they got on practising smooth and bumpy words.

◆ Brainstorm 'what helps bumpy talking?'. Children are skilfully led by clinicians' modelling into identifying the following: good breathing, light contacts, relaxation and pausing. Clinicians tell the children we will look at all these ways of helping over the next few weeks.

◆ Relaxation exercise.

◆ 'In the manner of' exercise. Children walk around the room 'in the manner of' a soldier, a puppet, a rag doll, someone on a beach, someone going to or getting out of bed, a frog, a tortoise, a racehorse, a jack in the box. Then they have to say their name/name of a friend/sibling/school and so on, also 'in the manner of' the word.

◆ Practice making 'tight' and 'loose' faces (for example, clenching teeth/relaxing jaws, pursing/loosening lips).

◆ Parents come in. A volunteer explains the session.

◆ Homework is given. We find 'making tension go away' a good relaxation exercise (Waugh 1991, p32) which can be practised by the whole family. This outlines a number of 'mini' relaxation exercises such as 'pretend your head is a ball and let it roll around on your neck. Roll it forward, backward and side to side'. Children can also be given pictures of mouth postures to practise with their families (for example, blow a kiss, look surprised, blow a raspberry, raise and lower your tongue).

Session 5

◆ Homework is reviewed. Children are asked to describe how they and their families got on with the exercises, who found things easy/difficult and so on.

◆ Clinicians use balloons to demonstrate the functioning of the lungs and how they fill up with air.

◆ Children have a competition to see who can take the longest amount of time to let the air out of their balloon (holding the neck between their finger and thumb, but ensuring air is continuously escaping).

◆ There is another competition to see who can take the longest time to produce first of all an *'ah'* and then an *'s'* sound on one breath.

◆ A final blowing competition – to see who can blow a piece of paper furthest along the floor in one breath. (It is important to monitor these exercises carefully. We do not want children to hyperventilate.)

◆ Children take turns to blow bubbles, using a gentle exhalation of air.

- All of the above are related to 'good breathing'. Children now practise good breathing by each saying a word, in turn in order to make up a sentence: person 1 says the first word, person 2 says that word plus another, and so on. The idea is for a breath to be taken when it feels comfortable to the child to do so, rather than for the child to speak for too long on the same breath.

- Introduction of pausing. One of the clinicians talks without pausing and the children have to guess what is happening. The exercise is repeated with the clinician this time using appropriate pauses. Children take turns to identify when they hear a pause being used.

- Brainstorm 'why do we pause?'. Aim to elicit the following reasons: to breathe, for thinking time, to allow the listener to take the message in, for emphasis and in order to make sense of what we are saying.

- Parents come in. A volunteer explains the session.

- Homework is given. Family members all try out exhalation on *'ah'* and *'s'* and see how long each sound can be maintained. The best times are recorded. Individual children work on trying to make their own production of the sound last longer and record their own best scores.

Session 6

- Homework is reviewed. Best family and individual child scores for maintaining a sound on one breath are reported on.

- Introduction of soft contacts. Clinicians converse with each other using both hard and soft contacts. Children in turns identify when they hear a hard contact.

- Clinicians relate hard contacts to stammering. Children practise making soft contacts using picture naming, starting at single-word level and working up to subject-verb-object ('SVO').

- Animal pictures are stuck onto the children's backs. By asking questions, using soft contacts, they have to identify the animal in question, for example, does it fly, how many legs has it got?

- Clinicians tell the children, 'We are going to make chocolate crunchies'. Clinicians ask questions throughout the process, for example, 'How do we melt the chocolate? What goes in next?'. The children must use soft contacts to give their answers.

- Summary round of how crunchies were made. Soft contacts must be used in answers.

- Everyone takes the crunchies they have made home with them. (NB: Ensure clinicians bring bags for children to put their crunchies in. We learned this lesson through experience. After making crunchies with a group for the first time and having no bags, we found a trail of ground-in crunchies from our rooms all the way to the front entrance of the hospital!)

- Parents come in. A volunteer outlines the session.

- Homework is given. Children use soft contacts to explain to their parents how they made the crunchies. If parents are willing, the children can make more crunchies at home as they explain the process.

Session 7

- Homework is reviewed. Children say if they made crunchies and how they got on in trying to describe the process using soft contacts.

- Introduction of speaking rate using the analogy of 'speaking gears' – fast, medium and slow – which compare to the gears used in a car as it moves from starting off to going fast.

- Clinicians demonstrate each speaking gear randomly and children in turn hold up a score card (1 slow, 2 medium, and 3 fast) to say which gear they thought the clinician was using.

- Each child is timed saying an identical sentence at gear 1 and then at gear 3, to ensure they can vary their speaking rate appropriately.

- On a flip chart, children brainstorm when they need to use slow, medium and fast talking gears in relation to particular talking situations. There are no right or wrong answers, as different children will view different situations as more or less likely to prompt bumpy talking.

- Role play. A clinician plays a teacher and asks each child a question in turn. Children use soft contacts to answer.

- Parents come in. A volunteer explains the session.

- Homework is given. Parents are asked to mark down on a chart examples of when their child has used the correct speaking gear in a speaking situation, for example, a slow rate when explaining something complicated.

Session 8

◆ Homework is reviewed.

◆ Clinicians and children together read and then discuss the story of 'Fraidy the Cat' (Waugh 1991, p28). Fraidy is a cat who misses out in life because of his fears.

◆ Group discusses what people may do if they don't like something (for example, peas) or are scared of something (such as a rollercoaster). Ideas are divided into categories – running away from/facing up to the difficulty.

◆ A clinician gives an example of when she faced up to something. Pointers are elicited from the children about what helped her to do this (for example, talking about the fear, getting support of others and so on).

◆ Children tell the group about any speech avoidances of their own.

◆ Children are given a chart with two columns: things I don't like doing/things I'm scared of doing. In turn, children identify one personal thing in one of the columns, preferably in relation to their speech. For example, a child may say 'I don't like answering questions in class' or 'I'm scared of taking messages'.

◆ Parents come in. A volunteer outlines the session.

◆ Homework is given. Parents and children together read and discuss 'Fraidy the Cat'. Children write down as many speech and non-speech ideas relevant to them on the chart outlined above.

Session 9

◆ Homework is reviewed. Children each state one thing they fear or dislike.

◆ Eye contact is introduced. Three sorts are explained – good, staring and looking away.

◆ Two piles of cards are put out, face down. One pile contains cards saying either 'good', 'staring' or 'looking away'. The second pile contains topic words such as pets, boys' names, or fruit. Each child in turn picks up a card from each pile and demonstrates saying the word with the chosen eye-contact style which the other children have to guess.

◆ Putting it all together. Children complete sentences (such as 'I like …'; 'My teacher is …') using a medium speaking rate, good breathing, soft contacts and good eye contact.

◆ The above exercise is completed using longer utterances, for example, describing verb pictures. After a successful attempt, the child gets a reward. (We use putting a sword into a 'pop-up pirate' game.)

◆ Parents come in. A volunteer explains the session.

◆ Homework is explained. Children are given a sheet with faces on, but with the eyes missing. The children have to ask 10 questions of as many different people as possible, using good eye contact. When they have done so, they can draw in the eyes on the pictures. They also complete a phrase completion exercise (fish and – ?; bread and – ?) at home, using the four features of good talking they have learned in the group.

Session 10

◆ Homework is reviewed.

◆ Two children go out with one clinician, while the rest stay with the other clinician.

◆ The two children who go out use their 'easy talking' to buy something at the hospital shop, ask for Speech and Language Therapy at the main reception desk, or give their name to Speech and Language Therapy reception (obviously this task needs to be adapted according to local facilities).

◆ The remainder of the children first play a picture lotto game. In turn, one child picks up a card and says 'Who's got an 'x'?' The child who has an 'x' on their card replies 'I've got an 'x'.' Next, the children feel and describe an object from a 'feelie bag'. Easy talking is used for both exercises.

◆ The children sit opposite each other in rows. A clinician reads out a statement. Each child in a pair gives an answer to the question to the child opposite, using easy talking. Then each child moves clockwise one place to answer the next question. The statements can also be found on Handout 4 (p205).

> **Handout: Sample statements**
>
> One thing I have changed about my talking
>
> Something I need to remember about my talking
>
> One thing I will ask a family member for help with
>
> One thing I could tell my friends about speech and language therapy
>
> Something I have enjoyed about the sessions
>
> One thing I am going to practise

One thing I like about my talking

One thing I did well in the group

One thing someone else has done well in the group

One thing I can tell my teacher about the group or about my talking.

◆ Parents come in. A volunteer outlines the session.

◆ Certificates are handed out.

◆ Individual follow-up appointments are made.

A TYPICAL PROGRAMME FOR 8–11-YEAR-OLDS

Rather than describe this group in detail, we outline some of the themes that we feel it is useful to include in such a group. Suggestions for appropriate activities are given in each section.

Group Gelling Exercises

It is important that any introductory exercises are not too threatening. If the children are asked to say too much at this very early stage, they may feel awkward and embarrassed. Conversely, they know that they will be expected to speak, and therefore may feel easier once the first words have been spoken. It can be helpful if such exercises involve action of some kind, which may take some of the pressure off speech. Games which do not demand that the children speak in turn may also be preferable.

Ideas for activities

◆ Children arrange themselves in a given order according to, for example, the distance they have travelled, the first letter of their name, their age, and so on. This involves a degree of talking to get the order right, and also requires movement as the positions are arranged and rearranged.

◆ Children sit or stand. A ball is thrown and the person who throws it says their name. Once everyone's name has been said several times, the game continues in a slightly different way. This time the thrower says the name of the person the ball is being thrown to. In this way names are soon learnt.

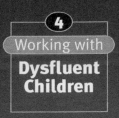

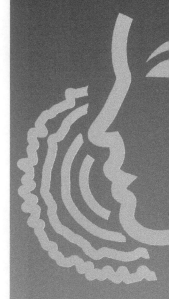

HANDOUT: SAMPLE STATEMENTS

One thing I have changed about my talking

Something I need to remember about my talking

One thing I will ask a family member for help with

One thing I could tell my friends about speech and language therapy

Something I have enjoyed about the sessions

One thing I am going to practise

One thing I like about my talking

One thing I did well in the group

One thing someone else has done well in the group

One thing I can tell my teacher about the group or about my talking

- A list is written on the board of such topics as pets, brothers and sisters, hobbies, best and worst lessons, favourite pop groups. The children mingle and find out as much about each other as possible, using the topics as prompts. In the big group, one child in turn is identified and the others share the information they have found about him.
- Children mime something they enjoy doing or are good at for the other group members to guess.
- People's bingo – described in Chapter 10 on schools.

Identification

We feel that in order to change, children, like adults, need to have at least some understanding of what it is they are changing from. The process of identification can involve brainstorming, small and large group discussions, drawing, listening to audio recordings, role playing, observation and listening exercises and games in the clinic, as well as home practice exercises.

Identification of self

The children identify their own strengths and weaknesses, the things they like and dislike about themselves, and how people differ (see ideas in our description of groups for 6–8-year-olds, earlier in this chapter).

- When looking at change, it is useful to look at things that can be changed fairly easily (such as hairstyles, clothes), things which may be more difficult to change (such as weight or speech), those which can only be changed at a price (sticking-out ears always seem to figure here) and things that cannot be changed (such as height or fingerprints).
- *Picture me* (Learning Development Aids) is a book of photocopiable pictures which can be used to identify more general information about the child. *Picture my feelings* using the same formula, looks more closely at identification of emotions.
- *ColorCards*® (Speechmark Publishing) present various categories of a range of pictures which can be used in a similar way.

Identification of dysfluency/stammering

This theme investigates aspects such as 'what is it like?'; 'how does it differ?'; 'is everyone dysfluent?'; 'what do I do when I stammer?'.

◆ Discuss 'what is stammering/dysfluency/bumpy talking?'.

◆ Use of audio recordings of different types of dysfluency.

◆ Checklists (for use at home) to spot 'normal' dysfluencies in family and friends. Heinze & Johnson's book (1987) includes several sheets which the child can use to differentiate between 'easy dysfluencies' and 'stuttering'.

◆ Cooper & Cooper (1985) used 'My stuttering apple' to identify individual overt and covert behaviours. 'Stop and listen' helps the child to identify normal dysfluencies in those around him.

◆ Rustin (1987, p36) presents a brainstorming exercise to look at the parts of the speech mechanisms involved in the child's dysfluencies. Each child then marks these on an individual diagram.

Identification of factors that might make someone dysfluent

◆ Discussions, perhaps using headings such as places, mood and content, are held to identify how these can all be factors in a child's dysfluency.

Identification of feelings about stammering

◆ *Sentence completion exercises*. For example, 'When I stammer, I feel ...'; 'I don't like talking when ...' (See Chapter 4: Assessment.)

◆ *Story making*. The clinician starts off a story about a child who stammers; the children each add a sentence in turn.

◆ *Role playing*. Children may be encouraged to express some of the feelings they have had by casting and directing other children in a role play. Such an activity is especially helpful when looking at teasing. The role play can be re-enacted when new ideas as to how to cope better with the situation have been elicited from the children.

◆ *Use of pictures*. Cooper & Cooper (1985) included a number of pictures in their sections on 'Stuttering attitude stimulus' and 'Speech situation discussion'. These outline situations that children may experience, and invite them to describe what they might be thinking or feeling. Children may also be encouraged to draw their own pictures of situations in which their dysfluency has troubled them.

Identification of non-verbal aspects of communication

The children are next helped, where necessary, to become good observers, first of others and then of themselves.

◆ *Observation exercises*. Several examples are given by Rustin (1987, pp76–77) of exercises in which children have to use or notice good non-verbal communication skills.

◆ *Therapists' role play*. Therapists enact a scene (for example, a vet's waiting room). They may demonstrate good or bad communication skills, which the children have to spot. Use of role play by the clinicians can be an unthreatening and fun way of approaching such a topic.

◆ *Use of non-verbal deficit cards*. The children are each given a card on which an aspect of poor verbal communication is written (such as poor eye contact, fidgeting). Each child talks either individually or in a group discussion, and the others have to identify the deficit.

◆ *Use of video*. Where appropriate, video recordings may be used so that the children can spot and rate non-verbal skills in themselves and others.

Work on General Communication Skills

Children are helped to increase their range of non-verbal skills in order that pressure is taken off the verbal part of their communication. Groups are an ideal practice ground for this type of activity. Specific ideas for this category of therapy have already been outlined in some detail in Chapter 6 on borderline stammering.

Reduction & Prevention of Development of Covert Aspects

We feel it is important that we approach our work on the covert aspects of stammering from two angles. First, we would hope to reduce any covert features that a child may have already developed. Secondly, we would wish to prevent the development of any additional such responses to the dysfluency.

The approaches we use include:

- Identification of 'hiding' behaviours through discussion, checklists, and so on. Cooper & Cooper (1985) used 'My stuttering monkeys' to this end.
- Problem solving, to finding alternatives to hiding. Problem solving is described in Chapter 7 on confirmed stammering.
- Waugh (1991) used 'Fraidy the cat' (outlined in our description of groups for 6–8-year-olds) to identify fears about stammering and help children understand that it is the fear that drives the stammer. Ways of getting the stammer 'out in the open' are discussed, using worksheets.

Fluency Control

Ideas as to whether fluency techniques should be introduced at this developmental stage and a description of various techniques have been discussed in Chapter 6 on borderline stammering. Rustin (1987) suggested that a variety of factors important in fluency are outlined and then children and therapist together look at those felt to be most useful for the individuals. Such an approach is more likely to receive the children's cooperation, as they will feel more personally committed to something they have been involved in designing. The degree to which children will need to be persuaded, cajoled, given control or suggestions will, of course, vary considerably.

Working on fluency in a group setting can be much more interesting than in a one-to-one situation. Activities can be more varied and more related to the 'real world'. In addition children, after some initial embarrassment, may feel less isolated as they use the technique with others of their own age and receive their feedback. They will also have the opportunity of hearing others speaking in this new way and of evaluating its sound more objectively.

Most approaches to fluency control suggest a systematic route from one word through to much longer utterances in reading, monologue and conversation. A variety of games can be used to introduce and consolidate practice at each level. Many of these are found in the programmes listed in Chapter 6 on borderline stammering. Materials used for work on social skills may also incorporate work on speech. The group is also a useful forum for practising skills while contending with both manufactured and real fluency disrupters (for example, background noise, interruptions, intolerant attitudes and so on).

Involvement of Parents

In the group for 6–8-year-olds that we have described earlier in this chapter, we have talked about how we invite parents to attend for the last 10 minutes of every session. The activities of the session are outlined, home practice explained and often the children present an example of a learning experience they have had; for example, speaking in a loud voice, using a soft contact. In addition, parents have their own initial session at the beginning of the group.

Groups in which parents attend alone can also be held part-way into a group programme. They can be used for the clinicians to explain the rationale behind the group and the type of activities which take place. Beliefs about and attitudes towards dysfluency may be discussed. Feedback can be given by parents as to their children's reactions to the group sessions and the things they appear to enjoy or not enjoy, and also about the parents' feelings towards the therapy. Specific topics may be introduced by clinicians, such as 'the conspiracy of silence', 'the value of praise' or 'turn-taking in the family'. We have found it useful to give parents a brief written résumé of ideas discussed in these sessions, and also of the main points covered in the children's groups.

Groups which are attended by parents and children together may be used for demonstration of skills learned and for children to 'teach' their parents specific techniques. Role-play exercises may be carried out. Individual needs and home practice tasks can be negotiated, and ideas discussed for practice during holiday periods. Review sessions can allow parents to help children voice issues that they may have found difficult to mention, and to discuss strengths and weaknesses of the group activities.

GROUPS FOR CONFIRMED STAMMERING

Working in groups can be especially important for children who are at this stage of construing. Their experiences of dysfluency can precipitate withdrawal from their own peer group, and bouts of anxiety and depression. However, despite these often acute feelings, we have noticed that there is frequently an accompanying lack of motivation; it seems as though the children acknowledge their need for a solution, but want it to be in the form of a 'quick fix', without the pain of long-term labour.

Benefits

Groups can be of benefit to such individuals in terms of:

◆ Increasing motivation

◆ Providing opportunities for peer interaction

◆ Reducing feelings of isolation

◆ Providing a safe medium in which to express anxieties

◆ Providing mutual support and encouragement

◆ Providing a safe situation in which participants can experiment with change

◆ Giving an experience of acceptance (irrespective of fluency)

◆ Giving individuals an opportunity to take on different roles, such as leader, supporter, helper, motivator.

Aims

A group programme for confirmed stammerers can focus on one or a combination of issues. Here are some suggestions:

◆ Teaching fluency-enhancing skills

◆ Modification of stammering behaviours

◆ General communication skills

◆ Reduction/elimination of avoidance

◆ Understanding stammering and non-fluency; the need for knowledge

◆ Desensitisation to stammering

◆ Development of personalised maintenance strategies

◆ Positive self-construing

- General social skills, including assertiveness
- Anxiety reduction
- Relaxation.

Meetings

Regular weekly group meetings can be a problem for individuals trying to keep up with class work, assignments and projects. While a session fixed to the same time every week can make life easier for a clinician with other clients to accommodate, it means that children miss the same lesson several weeks in a row. There is the added problem of explaining absences to peers and coping with return and re-entry into a class in progress. For these reasons, we have found it better to run groups for confirmed stammerers after school, in the evenings, during school holidays or towards the end of term. Our intensive groups tend to be held during the penultimate week of the school year. Little academic work is happening at this time, but children can still finish the term (and sometimes their time at primary school) with the rest of their peers. Non-intensive programmes are usually timetabled for after school or in the evenings.

We meet in a central location that has easy access to other sites (such as MacDonald's, supermarkets, bowling alley), as this can be useful for additional activities. In view of the typical age range of this client group, we think it is important to choose the venue carefully. Adolescents may get the wrong idea if expected to meet in a room with a Noddy frieze or Winnie the Pooh mobile.

Group Composition

Degree of dysfluency

Most clinicians would agree that the degree of dysfluency does not appear to be a significant factor in the group process of confirmed stammerers. Although we would concur, we do think it is worthwhile establishing, as one of the ground rules, how individuals prefer to be helped when they are experiencing severe difficulty. With one client in particular, we have spent several minutes just waiting, and we learned that it is better to establish a more productive regime from the outset.

If the degree of dysfluency is not a factor, then can the same be said about the degree of covert as opposed to overt symptoms? With this group, there may be some individuals who have developed substantial avoidance strategies, to the point where overt symptoms are hardly apparent. This may be construed by some members of a group as not stammering and, therefore, these individuals may be isolated and the group can split into factions or subgroups. In a situation in which there are significant differences in covert responses, it may be worthwhile spending time initially in exploring similarities and differences in individual behaviour, and helping the group understand the nature of each other's problems.

Age of children

As we have previously stated, the chronological age of confirmed stammerers may be wide ranging; however, many will be in the high-school and/or teenage years. Young people vary widely in maturity, and it is difficult to use age alone as a guide to grouping. However, where possible, we prefer to group 11–14/15-year-olds separately from 16–18-year-olds.

Sex

We prefer groups with a mix of girls and boys. It is interesting to note the group processes at work in these groups, especially the hidden agendas – matchmaking; playing hard to get; notice me please; do you like me?; I like you, but I really like your best friend better. In single-sex groups, we have found that boys can get rowdy, and girls tend to be giggly.

Number of clinicians

We consider that a minimum of two clinicians is required for groups of five or six members. However, with more clinicians or other helpers available, it is possible to have bigger groups, carry out a wider range of activities and deal with any individual problems that may emerge. Even with older children, we have learnt that it is advisable to involve more clinicians when activities involve leaving clinic premises; the unpredictable can and often does happen. Students can be particularly useful in these groups. Not only can they help provide more hands-on therapy, but they are usually closer to the young people's ages, and may be seen as allies who can understand them more sympathetically.

Involvement of others

While we are keen to involve significant others in the management of confirmed stammering, with a group of teenagers it is important to balance this with their own growing sense of self-sufficiency and need for independence. We must ensure, especially with this group, that decisions are made sensitively, in an atmosphere of openness and with full consultation, so that the adolescents feel they have control.

A TYPICAL PROGRAMME

The following is an outline of a week-long intensive programme that we have run for confirmed adolescent stammerers. There was a general theme of 'Me as I would like to be', and this was further subdivided into separate areas. We will discuss some of the activities which can be used under each particular area, rather than as a programme that stands alone.

Defining the 'Me I Would Like to Be'

Construing others

◆ In small groups, the children are given a picture of an individual and asked to produce some single words which might describe what they think the person is like.

◆ In the big group, children listen to a taped sample of a person speaking on a non-emotive subject. A brainstorming session follows, with the group suggesting single words that describe what they think the person is like.

◆ A group discussion follows in which we discuss how we make decisions about other people on the basis of how they appear/speak/sound.

Construing self

◆ Children are asked to do a drawing of the person they would like to be. Using the drawing, the clinician and the child together elicit constructs for each child.

◆ In a small group, we look at one of each child's constructs and discuss how you behave like that construct – how would you walk, what clothes would you wear, how would you behave with other people?

◆ Children lie on the floor on top of a large piece of paper. Someone else draws round their body to provide an outline. Children then write words on the outside of the outline to describe what people see from the outside, such as tall, smiley, long hair. Inside the line, children write words which describe aspects of themselves that other people may not be aware of, such as clever, sometimes unhappy.

Me as I Would Like to Be in My Family

Relationships within the family

Genograms The group are asked to draw their own family trees, using specific symbols to denote specific aspects such as permanent relationships, divorce, death and so on. In addition, they are asked to use different colours to indicate communication aspects such as talks a lot/a little, stammers/does not stammer, avoids/does not avoid with this person. Clinicians circulate around the group and discuss interesting features of the genograms with individual children. Volunteers are asked to share their drawings with the whole group. (The group can ask for elaboration on any items that are not clear.)

Role plays

In small groups, children choose to role play one of three options provided:

1 Negotiating going out by themselves
2 Negotiating more pocket money
3 Negotiating tidy/not tidy bedrooms.

Pairs of children rehearse, one playing a parent and one child playing themselves. The role plays are then performed in front of the whole group, and comments are made on how the child and/or parent can negotiate more effectively or a better compromise be reached. Reference is also made to individual children's 'ideal' constructs and how the child might behave in this situation, using one or more of the constructs previously identified.

Parents are invited to see a re-run/video replay of role plays.

Me as I Would Like to Be at School

Teachers' group Teachers comment on the child's pictures (me as I would like to be) and the ideal constructs which have been identified.

Children and teachers together compare their construing on:

◆ The child in the class now
◆ The ideal self of the child.

They discuss together which aspects of 'child now' could be changed to 'ideal self' and ways in which that might be achieved.

Pairs of children and their teachers consider areas in which their construing is different and how/why teachers see the child in different ways and in different situations.

More ideas are contained in Chapter 10 on schools.

Me as I Would Like to Be with My Friends

Sculpting A volunteer is asked to place the group members in physical positions which represent how they see the relationships within the group (for example, friends closer together/touching, vocal members in a more prominent positions), including clinicians, and, lastly, positioning themselves. Discuss any aspects which they would like to change to improve their own position, move to a more 'ideal self'. Repeat with several other volunteers, and compare the different sculptures that result. (This is especially useful with less vocal group members, as insight can be gained into how they view the group and the role they play in it.)

Ending Game

Feedback from the group Five of the 'ideal' constructs which were previously identified are written on a card, along with a rating scale. The card is pinned to the child's back. Each child then anonymously rates every other child in terms of how well they have achieved their ideal constructs. These are reviewed with each individual child, and targets/objectives devised for areas which he should continue with and areas which need further work.

SWINDON PRIMARY CARE TRUST FLUENCY PACKS

No chapter on groups would be complete without reference to the work done by the Swindon team (Claire McNeil, Claire Thomas, Beth Maggs & Sarah Taylor) and the Fluency Trust, which funds the residential components of the Speech and Language Therapy courses. We have already referred to this work in Chapter 4 on assessment. More recently, the Swindon team have produced comprehensive information about their courses, both in a hard copy and on disc. The packs (McNeil *et al*, 2003) contain outlines of three courses, of which the last two are residential. The courses are:

◆ 'Smoothies' (7–9-year-olds)
◆ 'Blockbusters' (9–12-year-olds)
◆ 'Teens Challenge' (13–17-year-olds).

Games for a variety of activities are explained, including warm ups, action games, and games for social, communication and fluency skills. Sample group timetables are provided for both children and parent groups. Each pack has simple, clear, well-designed handouts, to be used in conjunction with the course and appropriate to the age group with which they are to be used. The packs also contain assessment and outcome forms, which increase in number and complexity according to the age range with which they are to be used. Many of the ideas are equally useful for working individually with children and young people.

We cannot recommend these packs highly enough. Any clinician, however experienced, will find in them a wealth of ideas and information.

CONCLUSION: ROLES AND COMMONALITY

In all groups, clinicians should not underestimate the importance of practical details. Issues such as the delivery of children to and collection from groups, lunchtime supervision, safety aspects (especially when the children have been outside the clinic) and financial arrangements for travel and so on, all contribute to the smooth running of groups.

We have discussed in earlier chapters our belief that we must work in partnership with our clients and their carers and not adopt an 'expert' role. We are also aware when we work in groups with children that we are not 'teachers', although we are very often perceived as such. Children will, for example, show this by raising their hands to indicate they wish to speak, or asking our permission to go to the toilet or have a drink. We must make our roles and relationship boundaries clear from the outset. In this way these often embarrassing confusions over roles may be avoided.

Finally, the search for commonality is frequently present in the early stages of groups. Yalom (1985, p8) suggested that 'the disconfirmation of a patient's feelings of uniqueness is a powerful source of relief'. We find that groups help some individuals (both children and their parents) to be more open about their feelings. We can contribute to this openness by encouraging the group to interact sometimes without our direction. At times we are aware that we do not give children enough space to do this. We can be so intent on providing appropriate and stimulating activities and preventing boredom that we do not leave enough time for consolidation, for thought and for developing relationships that are valuable at any stage of development.

Between the ages of 3 or 5 and 16 or 18, children spend a large part of their waking hours being educated. The school exerts a tremendous influence on children, and if we as clinicians pay only lip service to the effect that this environment may have on them, we do them a great disservice. We know from many of our adult clients that schools can play a huge role in how they ultimately come to construe themselves. We have already looked in several other chapters at the influence that peers and teachers may have on the dysfluent child. In recent times, our work as clinicians in schools has expanded tremendously as we have realised how crucial it is to the development of children's sense of self and the way in which they learn to perceive their stammering. In this chapter, we focus on our relationships with teachers and how to work with them to help maximise the child's potential and ensure that the school provides an atmosphere conducive to the child's development of a positive self-esteem. We wholeheartedly endorse Gottwald & Hall's view (2003, p42) that 'the clinician's unconditional belief in the family's and teacher's abilities to be effective team members is crucial in the process of change'.

STUDIES

In the first edition of this book we mentioned various studies which demonstrated that stereotypical negative personality traits are attributed, by a variety of listeners (including parents of stammerers and clinicians), to speakers who stammer (Crowe & Walton, 1981; Yeakle & Cooper, 1986; Horsley & Fitzgibbon, 1987; Lass *et al*, 1992).

There has been further research in this area more recently, but no evidence that we can find to show that attitudes towards stammering have become more positive. Two more recent studies are worth a mention here.

That by Franck *et al* (2003) appears to be the first to deal specifically with the attitudes of school-aged children (aged from 9 to 11 years). The 75 children involved in the study were shown two video clips of the same 47-year-old man who stammered: he read a poem twice, once fluently using fluency-shaping techniques he had learned, and then stammering in the second reading. Non-speech characteristics were kept as similar as possible. Children rated the speaker on both clips. A 7-point scale was used to rate 12 bipolar adjective pairs relating to intelligence (for example, sharp/dull) and personality (for example, relaxed/tense). Findings indicated a statistically relevant more negative perception by the children towards someone who stammers, on all pairs except friendly/unfriendly and credible/not credible. In addition, the examiners involved in the experiment noted that the children's behaviour was different when viewing the stammered speech; for example, they often laughed and made negative comments. The researchers stress the need for education in schools about stammering, to address these negative perceptions – a view we would wholeheartedly support, and which we discuss later in this chapter. Franck *et al* also suggested that children who stammer could be involved in an educative role themselves with their non-stammering peers, describing this as an 'advocacy component' of their therapy. A study by Davis *et al* (2002) showed that children who stammer tended to have lower social positions in school than their peers who do not stammer, and were also more likely to be seen by their classmates as being in the categories of 'seeks help' and 'victims of bullying'. Although the numbers in this study were relatively small (403 children, mean age 11 years 9 months), its results are worrying.

Studies such as these have implications for children who stammer. If children are viewed in a negative or stereotypical way, such perceptions may well colour the expectations that teachers have of them. In addition, if children are treated as if they are, for example, shy or nervous, they can in time take on this view for themselves. If a lack of knowledge and understanding about stammering is more likely to be linked to negative attitudes, surely part of our role should be educative. We must therefore aim to assess a teacher's construing of the child in order to ascertain whether it is founded on an understanding of the individual as he really is, or based on a stereotype. We need to be aware that teachers' feelings and beliefs about stammering can have a huge impact on how they may deal with a stammering pupil in their class. If they have had personal experience of stammering in a friend or family member, their attitude to this person may well colour their view and the personal impact that stammering has on them.

SCHOOL VISITS

We are aware that many clinicians have long waiting lists and are under pressure to see as many clients as they can in the time available. Visiting schools can be time consuming. In addition, all too often, arrangements do not go as planned. The teacher one was hoping to see may be off sick, or has no one to cover the class, or has to talk to the visitor while simultaneously managing the class. At break, there is often no chance of a chat in the staff room over a cup of coffee; instead, the clinician may have to accompany the teacher on playground duty, where the conversation is continually interrupted by children, and the clinician and teacher are distracted. No wonder the school visit is often the first thing to go when we are under pressure.

Despite such difficulties, we believe that a school visit can still provide a fundamental part of our understanding of children – one of the pieces of the jigsaw that makes up the whole picture. We can learn about a child's interaction with others, his behaviour and general progress. Any problems he is experiencing can be highlighted. We can also learn how the teacher construes the problem and may be able to offer alternative ways of viewing it, if appropriate. We can supply practical ideas. If we identify problems within the school environment that we do not feel are possible to alter, for whatever reason, we may therefore need to help children learn to cope more effectively.

We can minimise the likelihood of things going wrong by careful planning. We try to book our appointment ahead of time, to explain the nature and purpose of our visit and to inform the school of whom we would like to see and what we would like to do. Ideally, a phone call can be followed by a written confirmation. In this way, it is hoped that arrangements for cover will have been made and the teacher will be prepared to see us.

Observation in Schools

We rarely undertake observation in secondary schools unless we feel we have no alternative way of understanding our clients or of finding out about their behaviour. Older children can be very sensitive to the reactions of others, perceived or real, and we generally feel that we best help the children in school by talking to them in their teacher's presence, rather than risk alienating them by our presence in the classroom. With younger children, however, we feel it is helpful to spend time in classroom observation. Whether we go 'incognito' or acknowledge that we know the children will vary between individuals. Many young children are happy that someone they know has come to visit them and will delight in telling their friends that they know us. Some others, usually the older ones or those with developmentally more severe problems, will make it clear that they would prefer it if their relationship with us is not acknowledged. We feel it is important to respect the individual's feelings.

Careful planning of such visits helps to ensure that the value gained from them is optimal. Adequate notice must be given, as well as an indication of how we would hope to organise our time in the school and what we might hope to achieve. If we are seeing a teacher who is coordinating information from a number of other teachers, we need to give time for this process to take place. With prior warning, teachers are generally willing to be very flexible and prepared to organise varied activities which require oral participation. Examples of useful activities to observe would be registration, circle time, literacy hour, group discussion and free play. We hope to learn two things from such observations. First, we can understand how the school day is structured and the kinds of demands that are placed on children. Secondly, we wish to understand how children cope with these demands.

Structure

We endeavour to gain some understanding of how the classroom is organised and of any potential problems that our children may be experiencing. The following checklist can be used to explore this area (Table 11):

Table 11 Checklist of classroom organisation	
Registration	◆ Formal or informal? ◆ Is there a set form of words to be used by all? ◆ Is there any freedom/flexibility in responses? ◆ Is there an emphasis on children sitting still and quietly when registration takes place, or can they move about?
Classroom atmosphere	◆ Do the children appear relaxed, at ease and happy in the class? ◆ Are there rules which the children know about? ◆ What happens when rules are flouted?
Routine	◆ Is the pattern the same each day or does it differ? ◆ Is there much group work? ◆ How are groups organised? For example, are they mixed-ability, or are children usually with others at a similar level? ◆ Are the children aware of any different ability groupings and where they are in the 'pecking order'? ◆ Do children's perceived positions in the class cause them any anxiety? ◆ How much time is there for free play, and how is it organised?
Teacher style	◆ How does the teacher relate to the children? ◆ How do children attract the teacher's attention? ◆ Is the teacher easily approachable? Are her comments usually positive? Does she shout much? ◆ How are children rewarded, and what are they rewarded for?
Views about to talking	◆ Are the children expected to discuss their ideas with each other or work in silence? ◆ Are all the children encouraged to participate in group work and to feel their contributions are valued? ◆ How are the more reserved or less articulate children encouraged? ◆ How are the chatterboxes prevented from monopolising discussions? Are children encouraged to be good listeners? ◆ How is 'difference' dealt with?
Other adults	◆ What is their role and their interaction with the children?

Table 11 *continued*

Pace of classroom	◆ Is there a feeling of rush and hurriedness – are children urged to carry out tasks with haste, or do they feel they have time to plan and organise themselves? ◆ Which is most important – the process or the outcome?
SATs (Standard Attainment Tests taken by children in state schools in England, Wales and Northern Ireland at ages 7, 11, 14 and 16 years)	◆ If the child is in a SATs year, what pressure might be placed on them to succeed? ◆ How does the teacher actually teach at this time? ◆ Is the atmosphere different at such times? How are the assessments carried out, and what pressure might children be aware of when either formal or informal testing is being carried out?
Listening	◆ Is there a feeling that children are expected to listen to each other in the class? ◆ Is there time for children who stammer to say their piece at a speed which is not going to put undue pressure on their fluency? ◆ Are children encouraged to speak about any problems or difficulties they are experiencing within the classroom, or do such things tend to be dealt with by another member of staff (year head, special needs coordinator, etc)?

The child in school

Table 12 represents a checklist that can be used when observing children in the classroom.

Table 12 Observing children in the classroom	
Entering the classroom	◆ How do children react on entering the class (at the start of school, after break, and so on) ◆ Do they greet the teacher and/or their peers? ◆ Do they tell others their news, or do they get on with a particular task, or seem unsure of what to do?
Registration	◆ Can children say their responses easily and when it is required, or are they dysfluent or hesitant? ◆ How do they react if they are dysfluent? ◆ How do classmates and the teacher react to any difficulty children have in responding?
Participation	◆ Do children spontaneously offer information and ideas during class discussion? ◆ Do they have to be prompted to speak? ◆ Will others wait for them to finish, or do they jump in if it takes too long?
Friendships	◆ Do children have particular friends or are they loners? ◆ Do they seem generally well liked/popular? ◆ How do they gain others' attention? Is it mainly through speech, or through other, non-verbal, behaviour? ◆ Are they initiators or responders?
Ability	◆ How do children seem to be getting on with the work? ◆ Do they find it easy or hard? ◆ Do they take time to start or finish it? ◆ How do they compare with others in the class? ◆ Do they appear to construe themselves and their work positively?
Coping with difficulties	◆ Do children ask questions to ensure they understand? ◆ If so, are these addressed to their teacher/peers, or to both? ◆ If they do not ask, do they end up doing things wrongly?

Discussion with Teachers

When we want to speak to a teacher, to whom do we feel it is most appropriate to talk? In a secondary school, this will depend on why we are making the visit. Perhaps we wish to find out some fairly specific information, such as how children cope in registration or whether they have many friends, in which case the form teacher may be able to help us most. We may wish to know about children's performance in a particular subject or with a particular teacher, who may therefore be the most appropriate person to talk to. If we want an overall view of children, the year head may be able to help us. If the Special Educational Needs coordinator has a role with them or is interested in getting to know them and collating information about them from a variety of people, then that person may be our best resource. If, however, they have little or no contact with the children then we might do better by seeing someone else. All too often, of course, we speak to the person who is available to see us! We also feel it is important for older children to be present during the interview wherever possible, to outline how the stammer seems from their perspective and to be part of any problem-solving approaches as to whether and how changes may be made. Looking at a child's records of achievement, including their personal profile, may be a source of useful information and a basis on which to build a discussion. In the primary school, we would always wish to speak to the class teacher, although there can be times when we will want to discuss a particular issue with the head or with a specialist teacher.

Almost inevitably, we will have only a limited time for discussion. In the time available, it is important that we relate to teachers as partners in a process that aims to assist us in our understanding of children and their dysfluency and in working together to try to find ways of helping them. It is all too easy, especially when time is short, to breeze in as an 'expert', bestow a few words of advice as to how the teacher should behave, and then breeze out! What a lot we then miss! For a start, we fail to hear the many valuable things the teacher can tell us about the children. We are constantly amazed at the depth and wealth of understanding and insight that teachers so often have about the children in their class. Also, unless we listen to what the teacher has to say, we fail to see how she construes the dysfluency, and we could be providing ideas that may be altogether inappropriate. Table 13 summarises what we aim to achieve in our consultations with teachers.

Table 13 Aims in consultations with teachers	
To understand how the teacher sees the dysfluency	◆ Are children seen predominantly as stammerers, or as people who happen to stammer? ◆ Does the teacher have empathy with how children themselves construe the dysfluency, or does she make assumptions based on previous experience or on inadequate knowledge of the disorder?
To ascertain how the teacher currently deals with children and reacts to episodes of dysfluency	◆ Does the teacher listen predominantly to content, or is the dysfluency the primary focus of attention? ◆ Does the dysfluency concern, embarrass or even annoy the teacher? ◆ Does the teacher 'make allowances' for the children or have lower expectations of them than of more fluent children? ◆ How are decisions taken as to whether children will or won't take part in a particular activity?
To find out how 'problems' are dealt with generally in the classroom	◆ Are they discussed with the individual or more widely within the class? ◆ Are they never mentioned, even if they are appearing to cause children concern? ◆ Is there a conspiracy of silence: children know they are having difficulties, so does the teacher, but neither party acknowledges it? ◆ Alternatively, is advice offered where a problem is not perceived by the children or their peers: are the dysfluent children advised to slow down, take a deep breath before speaking, and so on?
To gain an understanding of how children appear to construe the dysfluency in the classroom setting and to compare this with the picture we have already formed from our own dealings with the children and their families	◆ What is the level of dysfluency? Is the dysfluency seen to be improving or worsening? ◆ Does the dysfluency appear to occur more with some people or in some situations? ◆ Does the nature of the overt dysfluency change according to the situation children are in? For example, is the struggle behaviour more apparent in formal or time-pressured settings, or is speech less tense in a more relaxed environment when children have increased time in which to answer?

Table 13 *continued*

	◆ Do children seem to be aware of any difficulty in communicating and show any evidence of avoidance of words or of situations?
	◆ Is the teacher aware of any covert aspects of stammering? (If not, it may well be that a confirmed stammerer is construed as having less of a problem than if his difficulties were mostly overt. Indeed, without some understanding of the nature of stammering, the teacher may easily and very understandably assume that a child whose overt stammer reduces as he learns to hide it more successfully is either improving or coping better with his difficulties.)
Do other children appear to be aware of the dysfluency and, if so, how do they deal with it?	◆ Do they accept it, comment on it in an enquiring way or do they tease children when it occurs?
	◆ If children are teased, how does the teacher deal with the perpetrators? Is it similar to or different from the way she deals with other types of teasing?
	◆ How do dysfluent children react to any teasing?
	◆ Is this seen as an appropriate strategy?
What are the teacher's own speech behaviours?	◆ How quickly does the teacher speak?
	◆ What language levels does she use?
	◆ How much use is made of question-and-answer techniques in the classroom?
	◆ Can children predict when it will be their turn to respond, and how much preparation time they are allowed?
	◆ What general speech expectations are there?

Once we have gained an understanding of how the dysfluency is seen in school by the children and the teacher, we can begin to look at ways in which the environment may be changed to ensure that any problems children are experiencing may be reduced. Our observation and discussion may result in a number of possibilities for intervention.

Change the way we construe children

The visit may lead us to construe children and/or the environment rather differently. Observation may show us that child *A*, who is extrovert and talkative in the clinic, is withdrawn and quiet in the class. Discussion with the teacher may, for example, show us that the child *B*, whom we perceived as 'victim' is, in fact, the instigator of frequent incidents in the class. We may also have to modify our current approach to incorporate the new information. Perhaps we had been looking at listening skills in therapy with child *A*, but now our focus may need to change towards helping him become more assertive. When we work on 'teasing' with child B, we may need to help him to consider how others may be construing his own behaviour.

Help the teacher construe children differently

We may find that our construing of children is very different from the teacher's, even though the behaviours we observe are similar. For example, we see children's quietness as avoidance behaviour, whereas the teacher views it as shyness. It is important that we try to work with the teacher to understand how we are holding such different views, without a preconceived idea that we are right and they are wrong. Such a difference could, indeed, arise from lack of knowledge about stammering on the teacher's part or from a stereotypical view of the disorder (for example, all stammerers are shy). Providing information about stammering or suggesting other possibilities can enable the teacher to view the behaviour in a different way. Alternatively, we should be aware that we as clinicians may, on occasions, be prone to interpreting behaviours in order to validate our own construing of children, rather than approaching our visit with an open mind. We also need to remember that, whereas we know a child predominantly in a one–to-one setting, the teacher knows him as a member of a group, and the two may indeed be very different.

Provide information about stammering

In our experience, most teachers are only too pleased for the clinician to visit the school, and are eager to understand more about stammering and to know how they can best help children. In the inevitably short time which is available, however, we can only provide limited information. In looking at important aspects of developing partnerships with families and teachers, Gottwald & Hall (2003, p42) stated, 'For children to effectively use their fluency skills they have to believe in their ability to be effective communicators, and they have to come to terms with the emotional and cognitive reactions that may stem from their speaking difficulties. It will be helpful for families and teachers to understand that a realistic outcome of successful treatment is a child who communicates capably and with confidence. This outcome does not preclude the occurrence of occasional dysfluencies in the child's speech.' We would agree with this but take it further, in that we believe that developing and maintaining a positive attitude in children towards their stammering and to speaking should be our most important goal. In addition, we would endeavour to help children learn to speak as fluently as possible. It is essential, therefore, that this is as relevant as possible to the child in question. It may be useful to meet with the teacher, having prepared written summaries of our interventions, reports, future plans and so on for the teacher to refer to later, when she has more time to take in the information. Suppose our visit strengthens our belief that the child in question is still developmentally at an early stage of stammering. If this is the case, we need to look at providing some basic responses that we hope will help him to remain so. These could include ideas such as giving time, providing a good model, keeping good eye contact, assuming full participation and not intervening during dysfluencies. If the child appears to be at a borderline stage, we may look at some other additional strategies which could be useful. These might include creating opportunities for fluency or reorganising activities that highlight difficulties (such as registration) or which place children under time pressure. Children at the confirmed stammering stage may need additional help to become more open about their stammering, and encouragement to participate more in class.

We have found the 'iceberg' analogy to be a useful way of quickly and succinctly explaining to teachers the overt and covert aspects of stammering. This can be particularly useful for children who are developing covert strategies but whom the teacher may view as 'improving' because the overt stammer may be reducing.

Leaving reading material gives the teacher time to digest information in a less pressured atmosphere. The British Stammering Association (BSA) leaflet *The Child who Stammers: Information for Teachers* is a short, easily read leaflet which explains the nature of stammering and factors that tend to increase or decrease its severity. It also gives practical ideas as to how teachers can best help the dysfluent child in their class. Byrne (1991) includes a chapter entitled 'How Teachers can Help' which outlines the different ways that adults and children may construe stammering and also gives some general and specific advice as to how dysfluency should best be handled in the classroom. Conture (1989) attempts to answer some of the questions frequently posed by parents and teachers, such as 'Why does he stutter at some times and not others?' and 'Will continued stuttering hinder his academic success?'. Turnbull & Stewart (1996) includes a chapter entitled 'Stammering and School', which offers ideas to carers around such issues as choosing a school, and recognising and dealing with problems in school such as registration, reading aloud, and teasing and bullying. Another publication (Rustin *et al*, 2001) is written specifically for teachers and other professionals. It contains useful information on subjects such as what stammering is and answers frequently asked questions, such as whether children will grow out of it and what causes it. The book looks at stammering from an educational perspective and outlines are given on possible presentations of stammering and ways of helping in the early years, in primary school and in secondary schools. The book also contains a useful appendix of checklists (such as 'warning bells') and practical exercises.

Share information about the child

In our sessions with children, we often learn about things which it may be useful for the teacher also to know. Children may, for example, have told us that someone in another class has teased them, or that the dinner lady is very impatient with them if they stammer when speaking to her. They may have mentioned things about the teacher's own behaviour which are troubling them. Such issues will need to be handled with some sensitivity. Of course, children are likely to have mentioned positive aspects of others' interactions as well, and these should also be fed back, so that they are most likely to be reinforced. We have access to medical notes which teachers do not. We need to use our professional judgement as well as considering confidentiality issues when deciding whether any information from these should be shared. There may also be aspects of children's home life which either the teacher or the clinician do not know about – sharing such information may help our understanding of children and their behaviour. Obviously, when doing this we have to be aware of how the information became available to us and, again, need to be clear in our own minds about the boundaries of confidentiality.

Discuss alternative strategies – practical ideas

Turner & Helms (1991, p287) pointed out that ' teacher behavior directly relates to the student's self-concept and peer acceptance. Teachers appear to be in a prime position to serve as a role model, as well as a reinforcer, of children's social interaction. The examples they set, the tone they establish for peer relations, and the feedback they give to children are important influences.' When children are experiencing particular difficulties in particular situations, it may be helpful to work with the teacher to develop alternative strategies that can help prevent the dysfluency from developing further. In Table 14, we list some situations that commonly cause, or are perceived to cause, problems, and propose some possible solutions.

Teasing & Bullying

It is an indisputable fact that almost all children are teased at some stage during their school career. Teasing may relate to physical appearance (you are fat/thin/wear glasses/have spots) or to behaviours (you can't run fast/can't read properly/look disgusting when you eat). Children who stammer are obvious candidates for teasing, and for some this can be a serious problem. Dealing with teasing can be approached from two angles. In Chapter 7 on confirmed stammering, we looked at how clinicians might help children who are being teased

Table 14 Problem areas and practical solutions		
Situation	**Areas which may give rise to problems**	**Solutions**
Registration	Rigidity of format; precise form of words; short time-frame; attention on child	(Solutions should be the same for all the class, not just the child who stammers) ◆ All the class are allowed to answer using the words they choose (within reason!) such as 'yes', 'here', 'hello' and not be required to use the teacher's name ◆ Encourage children to experiment with different answers/use the names of different children in the class in their reply ◆ Children sit around the teacher as she calls out names. Teacher observes absence or presence while children count, in unison, the total of children present (unison speech tending to produce fluency) ◆ Children say a greeting in a foreign language, which makes the activity more fun for everyone ◆ Children give their answers while engaged in another activity, or approach and greet the teacher in their own words on entering the class ◆ Teachers will often create imaginative alternatives themselves once they understand the difficulties this situation can cause dysfluent children.

Table 14 *continued*

Reading aloud: It should be noted that reading in front of the whole class is a fast-disappearing occurrence in many schools, especially as part of the process of learning to read. In secondary schools it occurs for a different purpose, for example, as part of a drama lesson. In such cases, discussion with individual children can help clarify perceived difficulties in such situations	Uncertainty over words required to be read; being the focus of attention; feeling unable to read in a way which sustains others' interest	◆ Vary how reading aloud is organised according to individual needs throughout the class, to help children to gradually develop this skill and encourage an atmosphere of acceptance of different needs and abilities within the class ◆ For some children, advanced warning of a reading task gives welcome time for preparation; for others it only acts to increase stress ◆ Reading in groups or in unison can make the task easier ◆ Allow children some choice and control over areas such as when they want to read, whether just with the teacher or with others, or whether/how much to read in an assembly ◆ It may also be helpful for the teacher to discuss the stammer more openly with a child to let him know that she is aware of the fact that it can be a problem, and for child and teacher together to work out appropriate strategies. ◆ Ask the child what would help make this process easier.

Table 14 *continued*

Oral participation	Child's personality; self-esteem; negative construing of the dysfluency; attitude of the teacher and peers towards the dysfluency; response children anticipate they will receive	◆ Optimal participation is maximised in a classroom where there is an atmosphere of tolerance, where children's contributions are valued and where they feel accepted and helped to understand individual differences ◆ Rewarding children for content rather than fluency will make them want to 'say their piece', regardless of whether or not they stammer ◆ The behaviour of the teacher can influence the way other children react to the dysfluency. A teacher who listens and is at ease waiting for a response will promote this response in others.
Foreign language lessons	Lessons are, certainly initially, almost exclusively oral; teaching often starts at a time when children are also coping with all the uncertainty of starting a new school; difficulty in pronunciation of new words adds extra pressure	◆ Discussion with a child alone may help to ascertain any problems he is having and to find ways of assessing the progress of a child who participates little ◆ At exam time, a letter written by the clinician can go a long way to reassure children that their success will not be penalised by their lack of fluency.

to deal with their oppressors more effectively and/or to place the blame where it rightly should be, rather than letting the culprits determine how the victim should feel. In this chapter, we wish to deal with the teacher's response to children who are teased and also to children who do the teasing.

Response to children who are teased

Younger children will often report episodes of teasing to the teacher, who has then to use her own judgement to ascertain the seriousness of the offence and the effect the incident has had, before deciding on an appropriate response. It may be sufficient for the teacher to show a child that she understands his feelings and is able to offer him some reassurance. Perhaps she can help them to analyse the situation – what did the culprit actually do or say; was their reaction intended to be hurtful, or was it a (sensitive or insensitive) query, such as 'Why do you talk like that'? She may need to help the child to look at the most appropriate ways of dealing with the offender; for example, should they ignore them, tell them that the teacher will be informed, or respond verbally in some way? We would concur with many writers on the subject who propose that acceptance can be the most appropriate response to teasing (Van Riper, 1973; Peters & Guitar, 1991), but would suggest that this demands a degree of maturity which may not be found in younger children. Whilst a defensive reaction often provokes further stammering, admitting to the stammer often takes the wind out of the sails of the teaser: suddenly the provocateur finds he has nothing more to say, when his goading does not produce the desired effect.

Response to the teaser

We would suggest that, especially at a younger age, much teasing springs from ignorance, rather than a desire to be hurtful. Explaining a little about stammering enables the teaser to address their lack of knowledge and lessens the likelihood of teasing in the future. Suggestions that the teaser might actually be able to play a role in helping a child who stammers can also be useful.

Talking to the class

In some cases, it is useful to talk to the whole class in a relaxed way about stammering, but this should always be with the agreement of children who stammer. Young children have poorly developed empathic skills, and are often unable to understand how others are feeling. Explaining how children who were teased may have felt enables the culprit to see his behaviour from the other person's perspective.

Byrne (1991) suggested that, if there is laughter in the class in response to a child's dysfluency, it is often best dealt with in the same way as laughter over any other response, such as a wrong answer, might be. She stated (p46) that 'treating stammering as just another aspect of behaviour rather than something special and dealing with it in the same casual way is of infinite help to the stammerer and a useful lesson in tolerance for the other children'.

Teasing can be approached, too, as a general topic for class discussion, without relating it specifically to stammering. Nowadays, many schools have clearly defined policies on teasing and bullying, and there are established rules within a classroom as to how children should relate to each other. In some classes, children are encouraged to develop their own rules and ways of dealing with those who offend.

Development of friendships

It is our experience that children who have plenty of friends or who are good at something that gains them kudos from their peers (such as football) are rarely teased about their stammering. We do not advocate sending all dysfluent children to classes that develop appropriate skills, but we do suggest that consideration is given to helping children develop friendships if necessary. When asked if she was teased when she stammered, *A*, a girl of 13 who had strong and often unpopular views which she readily expressed, replied 'They wouldn't dare; my friends would kill them.'

Bullying

There are, on occasions, times when teasing cannot be contained, either by helping children who are teased to react in a new way or by dealing with the offender in some of the ways we have suggested. When teasing becomes bullying, we encounter something that needs more severe intervention. In the past 20 years or so, the topic of bullying has taken a far higher profile, both in schools and, more latterly, in workplaces. Schools are now required to have written anti-bullying policies. An anti-bullying pack, *Bullying, Don't Suffer in Silence*, produced by the Department for Education and Skills and updated in September 2002, indicated the importance the department has also put on this issue. (This can be downloaded from www.dfes.gov.uk/bullying.) In addition, *Bullying – A Charter for Action* was launched in November 2003, and all schools are expected to sign up to this document (downloadable from www.dfes.gov.uk/bullying/pack/CharterPoster_A4.pdf). Hughes (2003a, p10) reported that 'by the autumn, a £470 million behaviour and attendance programme will include general guidance to all schools in anti-bullying strategies, and specialist consultants to help local education authorities tackle bullying'. This all seems very positive for stammering children in schools and it is to be hoped that, as this information filters through schools, stammering children will be less likely to be bullied as a result. Over the past decade or so, the British Stammering Association has been considering the whole issue of schoolchildren very closely. In 1992, they launched their 'Helping stammering pupils' project, which aimed to foster cooperation between teachers, children and clinicians. Consultation meetings were held to investigate the needs of young people who stammer. The project considered how teachers might be better prepared to deal with stammering in the classroom, through improvements to teacher training at graduate and postgraduate levels. Bullying has also been researched at Sheffield University. The British Stammering Association has produced a pack for schools entitled *Bullying and the Dysfluent Child in Primary School*. The field of employment has been another area of investigation.

Children who are bullied often do not tell adults, fearing that, if the bully finds out, things will get even worse. If we have any suspicions that children we are dealing with are in fact being bullied, it is important that we act straight away and ensure that the matter is thoroughly investigated and appropriate action taken. In extreme circumstances, this may involve the exclusion of the bully from school. We talk more about dealing with bullying in Chapter 7 on confirmed stammering.

Hughes (2003b) looked at ideas that are currently being used in schools to tackle bullying. Clinicians armed with such possible strategies may be able to suggest appropriate use for some of these in the schools that they visit, according to the individual needs of the children whom they are treating. We list some of Hughes' ideas here:

◆ Specific problems raised as topics for discussion in 'circle time'.
◆ 'Circle of friends' – a skilled professional meets with the class, without children who are having difficulties being present, but with the knowledge of the children and parent(s). The object of the exercise is for the class to find ways of helping children and to develop a 'circle of friends' to support their class teacher in helping their fellow pupils.
◆ A 'buddy' system of support.
◆ 'No blame' approach with older children, in which the bullies are helped to work to support the victim. Hughes pointed out the need for sensitive managing of such a scheme, and noted that it is not something that experts have uniformly welcomed.
◆ A 'bully box', where notes can be left for staff. This could be especially useful where children fear repercussions if they report a bully directly.
◆ Hughes also mentioned two books on the subject of bullying in schools:
  – Thompson D *et al* (2002) *Bullying: Effective Strategies for Long-Term Improvement*.
  – Varnava G (2003) *How to Stop Bullying in your School: A Guide for Teachers*. London: David Fulton.

Talking openly about stammering

Talking about stammering may be useful for individual children. We would not suggest that the dysfluency is discussed unless the children are aware of it and also seem to be feeling some concern. If in doubt, we would advise erring on the side of caution, rather than risk identifying a problem that is not in fact apparent for children. However, if we feel that the children are troubled about the dysfluency, then talking about it in a relaxed way can be very reassuring. It can be very comforting and reassuring if the teacher lets a child know that she is 'on his side' and wants to help, but at the same time shows that she is interested most of all in the child's ideas and contributions. The teacher can thereby help the child to feel able to discuss any difficulties he is experiencing, and together they can look at the best ways of helping.

In discussing this very issue, Peters & Guitar (1991) mentioned that one of them stammered throughout their school life, but the fact that a teacher never once acknowledged it is described as 'very uncomfortable'. If the stammer is brought into the open, where appropriate, the conspiracy of silence may be broken and the child may feel less need to try to hide the stammer.

Outlining possible future developments

It is helpful if the teacher not only understands something about the developmental stage at which the child in question appears to be, but also is aware of any possible signs which may suggest a further development of the stammer. The teacher is then able to identify such things as struggle behaviour, avoidance, embarrassment and difficulties in particular situations or with particular people, and to understand their relevance. Any change in overall behaviour or progress may also be related to the stammer, and should be considered in this light.

Ensuring that you are easily accessible/arranging future visits

To derive maximum benefit from any relationship built up between teacher and clinician, it is important that the teacher knows where the clinician can be contacted if there is anything that needs to be discussed. Future visits can also be planned as appropriate, or it may be that the teacher can organise time for a visit to the clinic, if this is deemed useful.

Summary

In practice, of course, we must be aware of the difficulties there are for teachers who attempt to foster an atmosphere such as we have been suggesting. We know that there are ever-increasing demands on teachers' time in terms of administration and assessment tasks, and that staffing levels often leave little time for individual attention. We are conscious, too, that we as clinicians could very easily alienate teachers if we seem to offer ideas which do not take this 'real world' into account. However, we are also aware that most teachers are usually only too eager to help dysfluent children, and welcome any thoughts and ideas we may have to offer. By discussing these sensitively, with an understanding of the practical difficulties faced by teachers in their attempts to implement them, we are most likely to help teachers consider any changes they are able to make in order to promote children's sense of well being and maximise their potential for fluency.

SCHOOL LIAISON VISITS

Another development we have made in our work in schools is something we call the 'liaison visit'. Starting secondary school can be daunting for many children, but for those with a stammer who may have heard stories of teasing, getting lost, speaking a foreign language and so on it can be particularly scary. When children see it as useful, we arrange to go into the new school with them and for one or both parents to meet with the year head, the class teacher if known at this stage and possibly the Special Educational Needs Coordinator. Ideally, this visit is made as near to the end of the school year as possible, unless children are expressing specific anxieties that need addressing earlier. Children, parents and clinician prepare in advance the sorts of things they want to discuss, questions to ask and information to give. This will vary from child to child, and may include, for example:

◆ *General considerations.* Sets, languages offered, being late for school, finding the way round school.

◆ *Things more specifically related to stammering/speech and language therapy.* What happens if I am bullied? What do I do/say about speech and language therapy appointments? What if I can't say my name at registration? What if people don't wait for me to finish, or interrupt me?

◆ *Questions about fear around talking.* Answering questions, reading out or, surprisingly often, about not being given a fair share of talking or not being allowed to take part in class presentations.

◆ *Questions about areas we/the child may have not considered.* One child we did such a visit with raised concerns about the school bus, because he had heard that he might be teased. The teacher was able to help him with a practical solution, which was to get on a stop earlier than he would have done. Then there would be plenty of space near the driver. The older boys (the 'bullies') got on at the next stop and sat at the back. The child was reassured, and did not spend the summer holiday fretting. We usually bring up the question of supply teachers. Inevitably, they may not always be given information about individual children. One of the suggestions we have found acceptable is for the year head to write something in the child's planner which the child can, if they wish, show to the supply teacher at the start of a lesson, thus alleviating fears of how the teacher may react to the stammer.

We try to ensure that one of the teachers at the meeting is identified as a 'special person' for the children: someone they can go to if they have problems and to whom they can put a face to a name from the very beginning of term because of this meeting. We also suggest a meeting between the children and the teacher at half term to check how things are going. One of our clients, a very confident young man, was looking forward to high school and not anticipating difficulties. Nonetheless, he still thought such a visit could be a good idea, as it indeed turned out to be. However the idea of a half-term review did not suit him. There was a residential school trip just after half term and he wanted to arrange the meeting with his year head, who would be going with him, for a date after the trip. He anticipated stammering more during the trip because he would be so excited and he wanted to have the formal meeting with the teacher once she had seen his stammer at its most severe. We must never make assumptions, but find out by asking what is right for individual children.

Another way of preparing a child, or group of children, for secondary school is through reading material. Here we describe two publications we have found useful:

1 *Farewell and Welcome* (Cossavella & Hobbs, 2002). This book is aimed at helping teachers and parents to enable children to cope effectively with the move from primary to secondary school. It contains activities and photocopiable worksheets for children to use to help them deal with change in a positive way.

2 *Talking about Secondary School* (Black Sheep Press). This pack can be used by children transferring to secondary school and also by those who have already done so but are finding the adjustment difficult. Although it is produced with children on the autistic spectrum in mind, the activities could be used with most children. It comprises a CD which contains 14 scenarios each with four possible courses of action which may be more or less appropriate. It contains photocopiable sheets showing appropriate and inappropriate ways to behave in 14 different scenarios:

(a) Wearing uniform

(b) Forgetting homework

(c) The dinner hall

(d) The school bag

(e) Shyness

(f) The bus queue

(g) Timetables

(h) Homework

(i) Getting lost

(j) Showers

(k) After-school club

(l) Hard work

(m) Long way to school

(n) Bullying.

In addition, there are four subsidiary pictures of possible actions. An example on the topic of forgotten homework illustrates the format: the teacher on the main picture is asking the children for their homework; one boy opens his school bag to discover that he has left his at home. The four possible solutions are: running home to get it; saying sorry; taking a fellow pupil's work to pass off as his own; or making up an excuse. The pictures can be used for general discussion or role play.

Black Sheep Press also publishes an activity pack entitled *Talking about Friends*. Although this is not about the transition from primary to high school, it has useful materials for looking at some of the issues that children may be faced with about this time. Like *Talking about Secondary School*, it is also described as 'a pack of activities to develop situational understanding and verbal reasoning skills in children' and the different situations are presented in much the same way. A typical scenario is of a child handing out birthday invitations. It focuses on one of the children who did not get an invitation and asks how she feels, how the other children feel, what happened when you had a party, who did and didn't you ask and why. Four subsidiary pictures are then presented to the child who uses them to decide what the child in the situations should do (ask if she can go to the party, ask her Mum if they can do something nice on that day, get upset and angry or ignore everyone and sulk).

ORGANISING TEACHERS' TRAINING SESSIONS ON STAMMERING

Although training sessions for all teachers may seem a good idea, the practicalities for teachers often make it hard for them to get time off to attend. However, if they have a child in their class with a stammer, there is a greater likelihood that they will be released to attend such an event. Having said this, we should emphasise that clinicians must be aware that they may need to use all their powers of persuasion in justifying why a head teacher should spend money on employing a supply teacher for a day in order to release a teacher. Arranging for a group of teachers from different schools to attend can be a very time-consuming task.

In this section we describe various ways of running groups for teachers. First, we outline two typical sessions that can be run as part of an intensive group week for young people who stammer. Depending on the timetable for the week, we may ask teachers to attend for a half day or a whole day; we describe both possibilities here. Although we had thought we would get a better attendance for a half day, we have been agreeably surprised that the attendance for a full day has been about the same, with most children represented by a teacher for the whole day. Secondly, we describe a programme of in-service teacher training that we would take into an individual school.

Composition of group

◆ We have looked at compositions of groups according to numbers and ages of children in Chapters 8 and 9 on groups. In addition, we note here how helpful it can be to ask a teacher from both the primary and the secondary school to attend when children are about to transfer schools. This has several advantages. It ensures that relevant information about children goes from one school to another. It makes children feel cared about and that their problems are important and taken seriously. It also ensures that children identify the teacher in the secondary school as someone to whom they can take any issues about stammering. On the minus side, the primary school may often feel unwilling to send a teacher along if children are about to leave (we run our groups in July). If, in addition, the secondary school is also unable to send someone, children can feel unimportant and let down.

◆ Another point to consider is whether the sessions should be for teachers alone or should also involve parents and/or children. There are both advantages and disadvantages in the different types of group. Working with teachers alone gives the opportunity, and often the freedom, to address specific issues more thoroughly. However, working with all three groupings provides a broader perspective and allows more factors to be taken into account. In the groups we describe, parents and children are also invited, but opportunities are made for different sub-groups to be held.

Clinicians involved

A minimum of two, and preferably four, clinicians is required if sub-groups are to be set up. Ideally, both should know the children, but this is often impracticable.

Venue

In addition to offering accessibility and parking, the venue must have at least two rooms in order that group work can take place.

Day of the week

We have found that the Wednesday of a week's intensive course is the best day for teachers to attend. By this time the group has gelled, and parents and children have started to get to know each other. There are two days left in the week for clinicians to use the information gleaned from the teachers to inform the therapy.

A TYPICAL PROGRAMME FOR TEACHERS AS PART OF INTENSIVE GROUP PROGRAMMES

The following describes one possible way of organising such a group for teachers, parents and primary-school-aged children. The session lasts for a morning.

The groups outlined are both examples of groups we have actually run. We adapt our groups each year to the children who will be attending and the themes we choose to address. Generally, in a week's group, we will choose themes around self-confidence/esteem and social and communication skills.

Outline of Half-Day (Morning) Session

09:30 Introductions. The adults (teachers and parents) in the group are asked to introduce themselves and to say one sentence about the children they are with. The structure of the morning is outlined, as well as some idea of what is hoped will be achieved. The latter would include:

◆ Opening channels of communication between the three groups of people

◆ Understanding stammering, both generally and in the context of the specific children present

◆ Looking at problems that stammering may cause

◆ Discussion of practical ideas as to how stammering may best be addressed.

Handout 5 on page 249 is given out (but not discussed) regarding 'facts about stammering' (incidence, prevalence, possible causes and likelihood of 'cure'). Questions on these topics frequently arise and can tend to monopolise discussions; dealing with them in this way prevents these matters from taking up too much time.

The group then splits for the first time. One therapist goes with the teachers, another with parents and children together.

Teachers' group

09:50 Brainstorm what is meant by 'stammering' (as a forerunner to later exercise).

10:00 Talk by an adult who stammers about their experience of stammering at school. This outlines feelings, thoughts and behaviours of the person concerned. We hope that it also addresses the adult's perceptions of the attitudes of peers and teachers, outlines problems and looks at helpful and non-helpful approaches from teachers.

10:20 The clinician outlines how stammering may be thought of as an iceberg (Sheehan, 1975). Teachers are invited to consider their child in terms of their individual iceberg as it is now, as they think it might have been when they were 4 years old, and how it could be when they are 20, if the worst scenario is imagined. The clinician suggests that the aim should be to prevent that development taking place and, if appropriate, to return the iceberg to how it was at the earlier age.

10:45 Questions. We feel that it is important that the teachers have a chance to ask questions, although because of time limitations this session is inevitably very short. However, clinicians may not always be the best people to answer questions which relate to the practicalities of school life; in this case, we would ask for suggestions from other teachers in the group who can offer more appropriate ideas based on their own thoughts and experience.

At the end of the session, teachers are given a handout which summarises the ideas raised and offers both a general philosophy about how stammering may be considered and also suggestions on a more practical level. The leaflet 'The Child who Stammers: Information for Teachers' (BSA) may also be used.

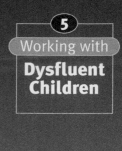

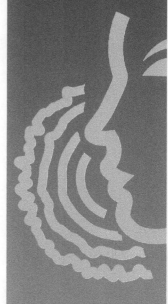

HANDOUT: FACTS ABOUT STAMMERING

Which children stammer?

About 5 in every 100

More boys than girls (probably 2/3:1 in younger children, with the ratio of boys to girls increasing with age)

Stammering often runs in families. Genetics probably plays a part in many cases

Why do children stammer?

We do not have an answer to this question yet, but research is advancing all the time

There have been a lot of theories put forward over the years, and it may be that there is more than one cause

We know that heredity can be an important factor

It seems very likely, from current research, that there are differences in the way the language is processed in the brains of people who stammer

Is there a cure?

The vast majority (4 out of 5) of children who stammer will not stammer as adults

Many will recover spontaneously; others with speech and language therapy

The older a child gets, the less likely it is that the stammering will cease completely, but the child can still learn to reduce the intensity of the stammer and its impact on their life

Parents' & children's group

While one clinician is taking the teachers' group, the other works with children and parents together.

09:50   Observation game – this game sets the theme for the session. We are aware that, when a family member stammers, it is all too easy to focus on that aspect of the person's behaviour and not to notice other things about the person. The game involves some people changing one aspect of their appearance. The observers have to identify the changes made.

10:05   A round of '[person's name] is good at …'. The theme is continued by this game, in which each person identifies one thing that their child/parent is good at. Again, the emphasis is away from stammering and instead stresses other aspects of the person. Both games treat the child and parent in the same way.

10:20   The focus now turns to stammering. A brainstorm exercise follows in which the group is invited to suggest how someone should react when children stammer. All suggestions are written on the board. The group then discusses the usefulness of the ideas and as a result some of the suggestions may be approved, others rejected or new ones discovered.

10:45   In pairs/trios, children and their parents use the ideas generated in the brainstorming activity to negotiate a mutually acceptable way for the parents to respond to the dysfluency. They agree to try this way of responding for the next week and to then plan a time to review it.

10:55   Coffee and re-forming of groups.

Teachers' and children's group

11:00   This session commences with a game aimed at both helping the group to gel and sorting the group into pairs of children and teachers who do not know each other. Cards are given out on which are written names of famous people, each of which has another half (for example, JK Rowling/ Harry Potter; BFG/Sophie). The group members have to question each other in order to discover their pairing.

11:15 Teacher and child pairs discuss 'times when stammering occurs and bothers me/the child in my class'. By working with a different child/teacher, it is felt that this discussion is more honest. The ideas are then fed back to the whole group and those that occur most frequently are discussed further. The group discuss the best ways of dealing with these problems.

11:40 In pairs comprising a teacher and the child from their school, the child is responsible for telling the teacher how he would like his dysfluency to be treated.

Parents' group

11:00 The clinician explains 'icebergs', outlining how much of what the children are now doing is above the surface and how our aim is to keep it that way.

11:15 Parents join in pairs and discuss tangible ways of trying to keep the dysfluency from becoming covert.

11:30 Ideas generated are discussed in the whole group. The clinician may, at this point, add in any ideas which have not been mooted.

Final session – whole group

In this session the focus is on teasing. If, as is most likely, this has been mentioned in previous sessions, members will have been informed that we will discuss it at this point.

12:00 Brainstorm any ideas as to how to deal with teasing in general (not just specific to stammering). These are then discussed and pros and cons of each are considered.

12:15 The same two role-play ideas are given out to groups of three or four (child/parent(s)/teacher). One idea does not involve stammering, but rather a child being teased for getting a low score in a test when everyone else has done well. The other involves a child who stammers as he asks to join in a game of 'tag'. In this case, the child does not play that part. The group play out their roles several times, experimenting with the most appropriate responses.

12:40   Issues from the role plays are considered by the whole group.

12:55   The morning ends with each member of the group in turn completing the sentence 'As a result of today, I want to try to …'.

Outline of Whole-Day Group Session

Here we describe a whole-day session. As we mentioned earlier, we have found little difference in attendance between half- and all-day sessions. Clearly, we can cover more ground in a day than in half a day, but we recognise that a session of this duration may not be feasible for all clinicians or teachers.

09:30   People's bingo exercise – see Handout 6 on page 253.

    Everyone – clinicians, parents, teachers and children – does this exercise. Everyone has a sheet and asks questions of enough people to have an answer for each section. Adults answer the questions with statements that were true for them when they were at school. Such an exercise has several benefits. It 'equalises the playing field'; the children and adults answer the same questions. It shows the adults what the children may be experiencing and shows the children that adults share some of their feelings, and that fears of talking difficulties can be apparent in people who do not stammer. Depending on time, some of the information can be shared in the whole group; for example: 'Did anyone talk to someone who got told off a lot?' Another way of feeding back is to use a line, on which participants position themselves physically according to their response. Taking the example above, everyone who is told off a lot goes at one end of the line and everyone who is never told off goes at the other end, with various degrees of 'told-offness' available in between.

Morning: Parents' and children's group

10:00   Small groups (parent, child, clinician) devise six questions that they will ask in a survey of people in the 'real' world. They think about who they will ask, who will ask which question (both parents and children need to participate), and where they will go to ask. Clinicians need to consider the advantages and disadvantages of children being in the same groups as

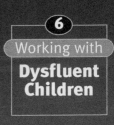

HANDOUT: BINGO CARD

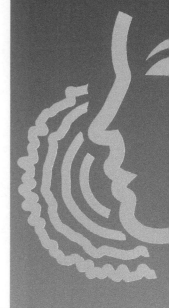

Would most people describe you as usually quiet or noisy or in between?	Are you good at spelling?	Do you like to answer questions in class?
Do you really enjoy maths?	Do you like taking messages to other classes?	Do you ever get teased about your talking?
Do you get teased about how you look?	Do teachers tell you off a lot at school?	Do you get nervous when you have to read out in front of the class?
		Do you ever talk to your friends when you should be listening to the teacher?
		Do you always do your homework really well?
		Do you sometimes tease other children?

their parents. For some, being with their parent can offer extra support and reassurance; for others, it may do the opposite and raise the child's fears and anxiety levels.

10:30   Role play asking questions, with clinicians introducing possible difficulties (for example, the person doesn't stop, is impatient, laughs, says something unhelpful or upsetting), and the group looking at possible solutions.

11:00   Groups go out to do the survey in the agreed groups.

12:00   Groups return. Parents are debriefed in their own group, facilitated by a clinician. Children are joined by the teachers and form a group. In pairs, children tell their individual teachers about the experience.

Morning: Teachers' group

10:00   We have been very fortunate in the past few years that Cherry Hughes, Education officer with the BSA, has been happy to join our groups and talk to them about whatever topic we have asked. Topics have varied from year to year. They have included the work of the BSA, Cherry's own experiences as someone who stammered as a child, the CD ROMs (explained in more detail later in this chapter) and, frequently, a question-and-answer session. Cherry has, in our experience, always been happy to talk on whatever topic is asked of her.

10:30   Coffee.

10:45   Clinicians outline overt and covert aspects of 'icebergs' in terms of stammering and the development of stammering (early, borderline and confirmed) (Handout 7, p255). In pairs, teachers talk about the children they have come about and speculate about their developmental stammering stage. They share their ideas in the large group. In this way teachers not only learn more about the child in their charge but also about the various manifestations stammering can take.

11:30   The information gained so far is related to the school situation. Teachers brainstorm how stammering may affect learning and social interaction.

12:00   Teachers join children (as above).

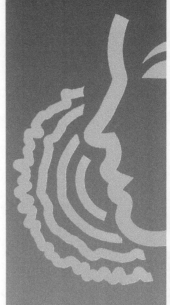

HANDOUT: DEVELOPMENT OF STAMMERING

	Awareness	Stammer	Avoidance
Early dysfluency	Child mostly unaware/ unconcerned	Dysfluencies, mild, unhurried, lacking tension or struggle, often consist of repetitions of whole words or of one or two sounds at most	Child does not avoid words or situations
Borderline stammering	Child has awareness/some concern, especially when actually stammering	Stammers may be tense and hurried. Usually, a sound or part of a word is repeated or the child stretches out or gets stuck on a word	The child may sometimes avoid saying a particular word or be reluctant to take part in a specific activity
Confirmed stammering	The child is aware and may think about stammering a lot of the time	Stammers may be very tense, with hard attack on words. They may last several seconds. Conversely, there may be little actual stammering as the child learns to hide the stammer	The child may avoid a great deal; for example, change words and/or avoid activities or situations. He may not make many friends and may shy away from 'talking' subjects

R Routledge
Taylor & Francis Group

Lunchtime: Informal discussions

12:30–13:30   LUNCH. Everyone is asked to bring a packed lunch, so that the discussions can continue informally. We suggest that participants sit in small groups of two children with their parent(s) and teacher(s). We find it useful to offer some prompts of subjects for groups to talk about, although some are happy to invent their own. Some of our ideas include:

◆ Coping with 'difficult' situations – registration, reading out, asking/answering questions

◆ Asking for help

◆ Presentations

◆ Talking about stammering

◆ Talking about the morning's activities

◆ Managing teasing.

Afternoon: Parents' group

13:30   Input by clinicians on icebergs and development of stammering (as with teachers' morning group).

Parents report back to large group for 14:15.

Afternoon: Teachers' and children's group

13:30   Game (we are fortunate enough to have a parachute and find parachute games are fun, release energy and, once again, are played on an equal footing).

There is a wealth of games that can be played. We have taken the ones we use from a book called *Games, Games, Games II* (produced by The Woodcraft Folk, 13 Ritherdon Road, London SW17 8QE). This is described as 'a co-operative games book'; it includes 22 parachute games. One game we constantly return to is a version of 'fruit bowl'. A clinician initially (and then volunteers) take turns in making suggestions as to who should change places. This can be done under, over, or round the outside of the parachute. Examples of ideas could be: 'everyone who had Weetabix for breakfast'/'supports Leeds United'/'is wearing blue'/'hates PE'/'doesn't like reading out in class'.

13:40 Children and teachers together produce an anti-bullying charter. This highlights the area of bullying, and gives children the opportunity to mention any problems they may have had and to discuss solutions which are acceptable to both children and teachers. A typical charter contains a list of rights, such as 'I have the right to be safe, I have the right to be who I am, I have the right to tell a teacher if someone hurts me'. It could also contain action points for what children and their teachers might do in cases of bullying.

Children and teachers rejoin parents for 14:15.

Final session: Whole group

14:15 Teachers, children and parents together discuss bullying and act out scenarios with solutions. We list some examples here:

◆ Someone starts to giggle when you are reading out in class. The teacher doesn't hear them.

◆ Someone takes your rubber from your desk without asking. When you ask them to give it back, they say 'w w w why sh sh should I?'

◆ You put your hand up to answer a question in class. You start to answer, but get stuck. Everyone laughs.

◆ Your best friend doesn't want to play with you any more. When you ask why he says the other children say you talk funny.

IN-SERVICE TEACHER TRAINING GROUPS

In considering in-service sessions for teachers, Bennett (2003) advocated a 'three *Es*' approach:

1 Engage – by being interesting and offering creative activities

2 Encourage – by praising efforts already made to help children who stammer

3 Empathise – by recognising the problems with which teachers have to contend (large classes, lack of resources and so on).

We run this type of group in a particular school on request for teachers in that school. To date we have run these courses straight after the school day, and generally have had about 10 teachers attend. We take with us BSA teachers' leaflets and recommended further reading materials. We also take with us copies of the CD ROMs launched by the BSA in October 2003. The relevant ones have been distributed to all English state schools, free of charge. It is important for Speech & Language Therapists in England to check with any school they are involved with that the CDs are readily available to staff, rather than stored in a drawer somewhere where class teachers have no access to them. One CD is for primary schools, another for secondary schools and the third for young people facing the demands of oral work for GCSE examinations. The CDs feature children, Speech & Language Therapists, teachers, and Cherry Hughes, the Education Officer, talking about their thoughts and feelings about stammering and offering useful practical ideas for managing stammering in the classroom. They are extremely useful resources that many teachers will find highly relevant.

Format of Group

1   Brainstorm what participants know about stammering. Clinicians then fill in any necessary omissions or fallacies. Usually, the areas covered by this section include:
    (a) Causation
    (b) Personality type
    (c) Incidence
    (d) Sex ratio
    (e) Possibility of cure
    (f) Intelligence.
    Sometimes, myths or stereotypes are raised in this exercise; for example, children who stammer are nervous and anxious/children start to stammer as the result of trauma. These are then discussed within the group.

2   Clinicians outline the development of stammering in terms of overt characteristics, awareness and avoidance (see Table 15). It is important that teachers not only understand the significance of an increase in stammer-

/stutter-like dysfluencies or amount of total dysfluency, but also understand the way a stammer may appear to improve when it is in fact 'going underground'. In other words, we need to explain the interconnection between overt and covert features and the various forms these may take.

3   Clinicians outline the 'stammering iceberg' and draw it on a board; teachers brainstorm overt and covert factors.

4   In pairs, teachers think of up to five potential problems which they feel could occur in school with a pupil who stammers. The areas teachers tend to come up with are the following:

    (a) Registration

    (b) Reading aloud

    (c) Answering/asking questions

    (d) Presentations in class/assemblies

    (e) The literacy hour

    (f) The school play

    (g) Teasing/bullying

    (h) Moving school.

5   Feedback to large group. Discuss as many strategies as time allows. We always stress the importance of setting up a dialogue with the child, negotiating performance opportunities, and asking how they would like the issues of answering questions and reading in class to be addressed (see section on strategies earlier in this chapter).

6   Questions (if time).

EDUCATING OTHER CHILDREN

In our dealings over the years with a large number of children and their schools, we have become aware that, although we may have been able to help effect change in the behaviour and attitudes of both the children and their teachers, we did little to address these issues directly with their peers. In this section, we wish to look at this issue by describing a strategy we have used successfully for some years now.

Giving Presentations on Stammering to Children in Schools

This idea was prompted by one of our clients, *P*, a boy of 14. We were discussing his stammer at school and he told us that it was always easier to speak to those who were aware of his difficulty. However, he still found it very difficult to mention, especially as his quite severe overt symptoms meant that whatever he said could take a long time. We discussed how we might help. It was decided that *P* and the clinician should meet with the year head and ask him to inform all *P*'s teachers about his stammer, so that if he took a long time to answer or struggled in reading out, it was understood to be because of the stammer and not because of a lack of ability. *P* pointed out that, although this might help the teachers to understand his difficulty, it did nothing to further the understanding of his peers. After much thought, the clinician and *P* together hit upon the idea of talking directly to the children. Initially, *P* agreed to be a part of this process, but later he decided that he would rather just be a part of the audience.

Outline of Presentation

The session described lasts about 25 minutes and involves two therapists. It can easily be adapted to fit in with timetable requirements. It may be particularly appropriate for such a session to be part of a wider course within the personal, social and health education syllabus. Follow-up work in class may be done by teachers who can address questions that the children may find it hard to pose to visitors. Strictly, only one clinician is required, but we would certainly recommend the moral support that two clinicians are able to give each other. Speaking to large groups of teenagers, especially, is a daunting prospect for the uninitiated.

1   After the clinicians have introduced themselves, a few basic facts about stammering are outlined (as in the School Presentation Sheet which follows this section). It is stressed that people who stammer are just like other people in all other ways.

2   Stammering is then compared by the clinician to having a broken leg. Usually, someone in the class has had or knows someone who has broken a leg, and what the experience was like. We elicit ideas from the children as to what it

feels and looks like, how it happens and how it is treated. A broken leg is visible, has an identifiable cause and will eventually heal; people who stammer, on the other hand, look no different and it is hard to see why it happens. They may or may not 'get better' in time, but improvement does not come by taking medicine or by wearing a plaster cast. Having a broken leg may inconvenience someone for a short period of time, whereas the effects of stammering may carry on. Children understand ways of helping someone with a broken leg, for example, by opening doors or carrying their bag; they tend to be less sure about how best to help someone with a stammer.

3   Depending on the age group we are talking to, we use short clips from one of two videos. Both are available on loan or to buy from the BSA. For years 8 and above, we would usually use 'A Voice in Exile'. We use two clips: one in which a boy is seen stammering while answering a question in class, and the other in which he is ordering a burger in the school canteen. On the video, some of the boy's classmates are laughing. It is likely that some of this older audience will also laugh. It is best that the clinician use some understanding in dealing with this. It may help, for example, to restrict her comments to the laughter that occurred on the video, saying something like: 'Did you notice how some of the boy's classmates laughed at him when he stammered? Often, when we laugh at someone's distress, it is because we don't really understand it or are embarrassed by it. We don't really mean to hurt the person, and perhaps we might be able to think of better ways of responding.' For children in years 7 and below, we use two clips from 'A Chance to Speak': one in which a boy is stammering when giving a talk, and another where he is being teased in the playground.

4   Pieces of paper are given out, and the children are asked to anonymously write down words which they feel describe how the young man is feeling. In our experience, children can be very perceptive and their responses often show a high degree of empathy. We share some of the responses with the class.

5   We then invite the children to consider what sort of responses they would like people to make towards them if they were to stammer. This is the most problematic part of the session, especially if it is a large group in which people feel intimidated about speaking. Returning to the analogy of the

broken leg may be helpful in stimulating ideas (for example, in considering whether to talk about it, getting a balance between helping someone out and taking away their independence, feeling concerned for them but not treating them differently as a person). We have also found it useful for us to role-play unhelpful responses if ideas given are either unhelpful or not forthcoming. For example, one of us might ask the other: 'What did you do yesterday?' The other will reply: 'I went to see a f...' and starts to stammer. The other person then tries to guess the answer and supplies words, 'film? forest? family?' and so on, before the person who stammers eventually blurts out, with evident frustration, 'friend'.

6   The session ends with a short tale with a 'hidden meaning' that illustrates the value of helping one another.

7   The children (and teachers) are given a handout on stammering and how they can help (Handout 9, p264), to take home with them.

School Presentation Sheets

Information on stammering

[The main statements we write on the board; the ideas in parentheses are suggestions of ways in which we have found it helpful to describe them. They can also be found on Handout 8, p263.]

◆   Five out of every 100 children stammer (that means that, in this school of *x* [number] children there are likely to be *x* [number] who stammer).

◆   More boys than girls stammer (we don't know why this is).

◆   Stammering can run in families (so if your granddad or Auntie Ethel stammers you might stammer too).

◆   It is very hard to change, no matter how hard you try (in fact, if you try very hard, it can make it worse).

◆   Stammering and stuttering mean the same (stammering is the word we usually use in Britain; they say stuttering in some other countries, like the USA).

◆   Some stammering is obvious (you can see it; we may demonstrate blocks or repetitions).

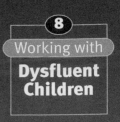

HANDOUT: INFORMATION ON STAMMERING

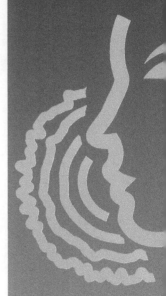

Five out of every 100 children stammer (that means that, in this school of *x* [number] children there are likely to be *x* [number] who stammer).

More boys than girls stammer (we don't know why this is).

Stammering can run in families (so if your granddad or Auntie Ethel stammers you might stammer too).

It is very hard to change, no matter how hard you try (in fact, if you try very hard, it can make it worse).

Stammering and stuttering mean the same (stammering is the word we usually use in Britain; they say stuttering in some other countries, like the USA).

Some stammering is obvious (you can see it; we may demonstrate blocks or repetitions).

Some stammering is not obvious (people try to hide it; example of wanting a Mars bar and coming out of the shop with a Flake instead).

People who stammer are the same as everyone else in other ways (just as sporty, intelligent, good looking, artistic, interesting and so on – or not – as any one else).

Many famous people stammer (use guessing games to help children elicit, for example, a famous prime minister in the war [Churchill], a King of England [George VI], a pop idol [Gareth Gates], a film actor [Bruce Willis] the actor who plays Mr Bean [Rowan Atkinson]).

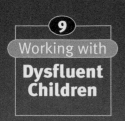
HANDOUT: STAMMERING – SOME QUESTIONS ANSWERED

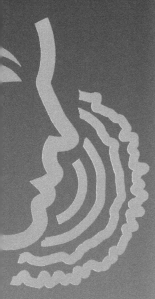

What is stammering?

◆ Stammering is talking that is bumpy, repeated, tense or jerky.

◆ Sometimes people try to hide it. They may say a different word from the one they want to (like 'Flake' instead of 'Mars bar'). They may not do things they really want to do (like answer a question in class).

◆ Stammering can make people feel really sad or frustrated.

Who stammers?

◆ Five in every 100 children stammer.

◆ More boys than girls stammer.

◆ Anyone can have a stammer – people who stammer are just as clever, artistic, sporty, clumsy, nervous, confident and so on as anyone else.

◆ Many famous people stammer.

What should I do to help someone who stammers?

◆ Look at them when you talk (like you do with anyone else). It is really hard for people when you look around or at the floor. It can make them feel you are not interested.

◆ Give the person your full attention, just as you would with anyone.

◆ Give the person time to say what they want; don't interrupt them or guess what they are saying.

◆ Be there for them if they want to talk about their stammer.

◆ Don't laugh or ridicule them when they stammer, and stick up for them if anyone else does this.

◆ Don't talk really quickly, so they feel they have to do so as well.

Most importantly

◆ Be interested in WHAT the person is saying, not HOW they are saying it.

◆ Some stammering is not obvious (people try to hide it; example of wanting a Mars bar and coming out of the shop with a Flake instead).

◆ People who stammer are the same as everyone else in other ways (just as sporty, intelligent, good looking, artistic, interesting and so on – or not – as any one else).

◆ Many famous people stammer (use guessing games to help children elicit, for example, a famous prime minister in the war [Churchill], a King of England [George VI], a pop idol [Gareth Gates], a film actor [Bruce Willis] the actor who plays Mr Bean [Rowan Atkinson]).

The story

First explain to the children that this is a story with a 'meaning'. Ask them to think about what the meaning might be and to tell us at the end.

There was once a place called Hell. It may surprise you to know that Hell was a beautiful place, in a garden full of wonderful trees and flowers. In the middle of the garden was a building called a pagoda in which there was a huge hall. In the hall was a huge dining table and on the table was every sort of delicious food you could ever imagine (ask the children about the favourite foods they would have there). There was, however, a rule in Hell about the food. You could only eat it with chopsticks 3 metres long. (Pause to let the children work out what this means; younger children may need the clinician to demonstrate visually.)

Heaven, meanwhile, was also a beautiful place, in a garden with the same wonderful trees and flowers, the same pagoda, the same hall and the same food. (Ask the children to remember some of the food they elicited.) The same rule about eating the food also existed in Heaven.

The difference between Hell and Heaven is that, in Heaven, the people learned to feed each other.

We then ask the children for the 'moral' or 'meaning' of the story. In our experience to date someone has always come up with the 'right' answer – that it is important to help other people. We then relate this to our own problems and to a child with a stammer. If we help each other, we usually cope much better with our problems.

Points to Consider

◆ *Gaining permission* We feel it is essential that we only do such a presentation if our clients see it as something that will be of personal benefit. There should be no coercion!

◆ *Children's involvement* Recently, we have asked some of our clients if they would like to be involved in such a group. Usually, we get a negative response. Occasionally, however, we find children want to be identified as having a stammer or even to take a more pro-active role, such as explaining something about stammering in general, or more specifically as it relates to their own experience. We, of course, encourage such participation, but make it clear that children can change their minds at any point in terms of participating at all or changing the way in which they participate.

◆ *Numbers present*. Too large a group may be inhibiting for children and clinicians alike, and prevent people from volunteering. We rarely now do this presentation to more than one class at a time.

◆ *Type of group*. This type of presentation can sit very comfortably in the personal, health and social education curriculum. After some unhelpful experiences with older children, we now consider the 7–11 year age group to be the most suitable and rarely present to young people over the age of 12.

CONCLUSION

Clinicians have recognised for many years the importance of working with parents of children who stammer. In the last ten years they have also considered it essential to work with schools, where children spend a large part of their day. If we are able to affect the understanding of children towards stammering, we not only may be alleviating some of the problems that children currently experience, but also may be affecting those who will be the citizens of the future.

We hope this partnership with teachers will continue to develop and further increase the help available for dysfluent children.

Chapter 11: Outcomes

OVERVIEW

Outcomes are important in any therapeutic intervention, not least stammering. We believe that this is an appropriate topic for a concluding chapter, as it allows us to summarise what we believe to be the key components of the management of dysfluent children. Outcomes have important links to efficacy and theory. For example, by looking at the outcomes of our therapy and comparing these with our initial aims, we are able to determine whether or not we have been effective. Then, in terms of theory, any consideration of outcome and/or efficacy reflects a theoretical understanding of stammering. If, for example, we believe that stammering is a one-dimensional, behavioural problem, then our outcome measures will focus on the quantitative assessment of the overt symptoms of stammering, and efficacy will relate to the alleviation or elimination of these behaviours. Readers will, by this point in the text, understand that we see stammering as multifactoral, and so our outcomes relate to the management of the entire range of issues and the implications of stammering for the child and his family. This is a view that has been echoed by others. For example, in 2002 a group of 'scientists and consumers' in stammering met in America and, among a range of topics, discussed outcomes. In their summary report (Yaruss & Reeves, 2002), they concluded that any consideration of outcomes should include:

◆ The perspective of both the client and the family

◆ Assessment of the client's communication attitudes

◆ Consideration of personal stories and narratives

◆ Incorporation of self-assessment in the treatment evaluation process.

There has been some discussion of outcome measures in relation to the particular theoretical multifactorial model that we have discussed in this text (demands and capacities). Yaruss (2005) has argued that the adoption of a multifactorial approach means that stammering should be seen as 'an inherent difficulty with the child's language and motor systems'. This also implies that therapy and the subsequent evaluation of outcomes may relate to a range of aspects of the problem, rather than purely 'surface behaviours'.

From this perspective, Manning (2001) focused on treatment and summarised the process as follows:

◆ Improving a child's capacity for producing fluent speech
◆ Reducing environmental responses to fluency-disrupting stimuli (or desensitising the speaker to stimuli that cannot be reduced or eliminated).

Manning stated this is achieved through enhancing the child's enjoyment of speaking and empowering the child to understand and use speech-controlling techniques. He went on to advocate that these techniques should 'achieve and expand fluency'. Through this treatment process, he believes, the child's self-confidence as a speaker and a person improves, and this would include the management of teasing/bullying as required.

In 2004 Yaruss made a number of suggestions to help clinicians evaluate therapeutic outcomes. He suggested (pp49–57) that clinicians should:

1 Work with the client to determine the specific goals of treatment:
   (a) Develop a rapport
   (b) Empower the client to make choices in treatment (and in life in general)
   (c) Listen to the client and not impose on the client their own beliefs about stammering
   (d) Give the client the opportunity to develop and grow during the course of treatment.

2 Not assume or require that all clients achieve the same outcome.

3 Collect meaningful baseline data and continue to collect data throughout treatment.

4 Collect data in multiple situations, both in and out of clinic.

5 Collect data about more than just speech fluency.

6 Not be fooled by the variability of stuttering.

7 Not let the client be fooled by the variability of stuttering.

8 Remember that the published, empirical literature on stuttering is not yet complete.

A TEN-POINT PLAN FOR OUTCOMES

When we consider what our criteria are for evaluating outcomes, a number of key elements come to mind. These summarise much of what we have discussed in this text. However, here we have tried to pull together the elements which are pertinent to all the stages of fluency that we have described. In addition to listing our ten elements, we include a sample of ideas which reflect how these outcomes might be achieved.

1 Reduced Anxiety in the Child and those in his Environment

This can be achieved in a variety of ways, such as:

◆ Giving information to carers and other professionals regarding management of the problem specific to their situation

◆ Identifying and addressing their particular concerns, including their worst possible scenarios and the 'what ifs'

◆ Creating a dialogue between the child and these others

◆ Creating a dialogue between the speech & language therapist and family and school/nursery

◆ Speech & language therapist acting as a resource for child, family, school, and so on, so that they know where to come in the future.

2 Empower the Child

Examples of ways in which this can be achieved are as follows:

◆ Ask the child. Involve him in decision-making processes in his own management and in clinic issues, including giving him the choice of what, if any, fluency strategies might be used

◆ Encourage the family and other professionals to adopt the approach of involving the child in decision making

◆ Have the child meet other children in the same or similar situation

- Listen to the child
- When asking a child his opinion, don't accept a 'don't know' response unless you are convinced he really does not know
- Model making choices in clinic
- Teach the family negotiation skills
- Help the child's voice to be heard
- Foster in the home environment an open attitude to others' opinions.

3 Empower the Parents/Carers

The following are ideas for achieving this outcome:

- Give information on stammering and its implications
- Listen to the parents'/carers' current and future concerns and address them
- Believe what they say about the child's fluency outside the clinic
- Teach problem-solving skills
- Have them meet other families who are in a similar situation
- Negotiate targets with the family, with a review date – that is, give them something to *do*
- Facilitate communication between the family and the child.

4 Develop Fluency Strategies Where Possible

This can be achieved in a variety of ways, such as:

- Start from what the child can do (that is, the point at which he is fluent)
- Teach fluency strategies (for example, rate control, easy onset, smooth speech)
- Teach communication skills (for example, eye contact, positive body language)
- Facilitate a positive attitude to communication in the home
- Facilitate a positive attitude to communication in school, especially with regard to situations that the child finds difficult
- Encourage the family to use an appropriate language level and reduce other demands in order to promote more fluency in the child (for example, good turn-taking in the family, reduced time pressure, reduced demand for speech)

In young children, encourage the family to establish an individual 'talking time' with the child in which they use several strategies to facilitate his fluency. This is especially helpful in a busy household, where there is lots of competition and when the child is having a more dysfluent phase.

5 Desensitise the Child to Stammering

Here are some ways in which this might be achieved:

◆ Encourage openness in the child
◆ Promote an open attitude about stammering and speaking in general in the home and other situations in which the child experiences dysfluent speech
◆ Teach the child use of voluntary stammering, if appropriate
◆ Use situational hierarchies to encourage the child to 'risk' speaking in difficult situations.

6 Reduced Avoidance/Limited Development of Avoidance Behaviours

Here are some ideas for achieving this outcome:

◆ Facilitate the child's monitoring of any avoidances (sound, word, situation, relationship, and so on)
◆ Facilitate the family's monitoring of any avoidance, if appropriate, and with the child's agreement
◆ Encourage the child to say a word that he has changed
◆ Encourage the child to participate in situations he avoids, using a supported approach
◆ Help the child work through a hierarchy of avoided situations
◆ Make the teacher aware of avoidance as a possible response in school situations, and help her manage this in a supportive manner
◆ Encourage the child to take risks when opportunities are presented
◆ Have other family members acknowledge any situations they find difficult and/or avoid. Encourage the child to take an active role in helping them reduce their own avoidance.

7 Increased Confidence and Self-Esteem

This outcome might be achieved in several ways. Here are some examples:

◆ Facilitate the use of praise in the home for speech and non-speech behaviours as appropriate

◆ Introduce reward systems such as star charts

◆ Encourage the use of supported risk-taking behaviour ('having a go') in the home generally and in the child in particular

◆ Encourage carers/family members to point out to the child things he is particularly good at

◆ Encourage participation in activities the child is good at and enjoys, which may or may not require speaking skills (for example, drama, sports such as swimming)

◆ Encourage the child to acknowledge his strengths, for example, through use of reflective diaries, dialogue at home, records of achievements

◆ Help the child seek out feedback from others who would be supportive of his efforts

◆ Encourage a home environment where it is acceptable to 'have a go' and fail.

8 Creation of a Supportive Network

Some ideas for achieving this outcome are as follows:

◆ Encourage the child to join a group of other children who stammer

◆ Encourage the parents to join a group of other parents with children who are dysfluent

◆ Put the child and family in touch with the British Stammering Association or other equivalent self-help organisation

◆ Encourage the child to bring a friend along to a speech and language therapy session, so they can support the child in working on particular targets and/or behaviours

◆ Suggest to the family that they encourage the child to bring special friends home to play/have tea/for a sleep-over.

9 Develop an Honest, Open Relationship

The following are several ways in which this might be achieved:

◆ Be realistic about the outcomes of therapy (but don't take away hope)

◆ Don't make false promises

◆ Don't collude with family members

◆ Involve the child in any decision-making process

◆ Always be clear about what information and/or attitudes that the child has reported in therapy will to be passed on to others

◆ Use self-disclosure appropriately

◆ Report to the child the outcomes of any discussions with other professionals which take place in his absence (for example, after a school visit).

10 Teach Dynamic Skills

Our clinical work has shown that, in order to maximise long-term outcomes, our management should include teaching of skills that would be responsive to the child's needs both in the present and in the future. We acknowledge that we cannot always predict what the child might need in 6 months' time, but there are some skills which can help the child to be his own therapist. Here are some examples of what we consider to be skills that would facilitate this process:

◆ Problem solving in self

◆ Problem solving in the family

◆ Praise/reinforcement in others

◆ Ability to self-reinforce

◆ Negotiation skills in the family

◆ Self-monitoring of speech strategies

◆ Self-monitoring of avoidance behaviours

◆ Good communication skills

◆ Positive self-esteem and self-image.

CONCLUDING REMARKS

In considering the measurement of efficacy for this client group, one is struck by the wide range of possible outcomes which exist. At one level, we have the possibility of promoting fluent speech in very young children and creating an environment which is conducive to its maintenance. Then, at the other end of the spectrum, we would consider the achievement of overt, controlled stammering, reduced avoidance behaviours and desensitisation to stammering as a positive outcome for an adolescent.

Our 10-point plan is an overview of possible outcomes from which a therapist might select. The balance and choice she makes will depend ultimately on what she sees as the child's and family's needs at the time of assessment. However, the therapist will be flexible and responsive to other issues that emerge over the course of therapy, adding or removing elements as appropriate.

Finally, we would like to share something from our work with adults who stammer. Often, in sessions with both individuals and groups of adults, we will ask clients to draw their stammer. Over a number of years we have had a variety of responses, but no one drawing has been the same as any other. When we look at the vast array of representations, we cannot help but be struck by the insight they reveal of what a devastating problem stammering can become. An apparently simple difficulty in speech fluency can distort and twist the client's view of the world, often appearing as a great burden that they shoulder and with which they face impossible odds.

Our role must be to convince individuals who visit our clinics that the burden is not theirs to pick up. They can examine it critically, perhaps define its constituent parts, but they should not regard it as belonging to them. It must remain detached from them and not slow or limit their growth or progress through life.

For those young clients who come through the door of our clinic and who we know have already lifted the burden of stammering onto their shoulders, our aim should be to create some way of reducing the burden and dissipating its contents. Ultimately, we hope that their burden will be light enough for them to follow their chosen path without hindrance and allow them to fulfil their potential.

Bibliography

Adams MR, 1990, 'The demands and capacities model 1: Theoretical elaborations', *Journal of Fluency Disorders* 15, pp135–41.

Ambrose N & Yairi E, 1995, 'The role of repetition units in the differential diagnosis of early childhood incipient stuttering', *American Journal of Speech & Language Pathology* 4, pp82–88.

Ambrose N & Yairi E, 1999, 'Normative data for early childhood stammering', *Journal of Speech Language & Hearing Research* 42, pp895–909.

Andre S & Guitar B, 1979, *A-19 Scale for children who stammer*, University of Vermont, Burlington, VT.

Andrews G & Craig A, 1988, 'Prediction of outcome after treatment for stuttering', *British Journal of Psychiatry* 153, pp236–40.

Andrews G & Harris M, 1964, *The Syndrome of Stuttering*, Heinemann Books, London.

Bannister A, 2002, 'Setting the scene: Child development and the use of action methods', Bannister A & Huntington A (eds), *Communicating with Children and Adolescents: Action for Change*, Jessica Kingsley, London.

Bardrick RA & Sheehan JG, 1956, 'Emotional loading as a source of conflict in stuttering', *American Psychologist* 11, p391.

Bennett EM, 2003, 'Planning a teacher in-service programe for stuttering disorders', *Seminars in Speech and Language* 24 (1), pp53–58.

Benson JF, 1987, *Working Together Creatively with Groups*, Tavistock Publications, London.

Bernstein-Ratner N, Rooney B & Macwhinney B, 1996, 'Analysis of stuttering using CHILDES and CLAN', *Clinical Linguistics & Phonetics* 10, pp167–87.

Bloodstein O, 1970, 'Stuttering and normal nonfluency: a continuity hypothesis', *British Journal of Disorders of Communication* 5, pp30–39.

Bloodstein O, 1974, 'The rules of early stuttering', *Journal of Speech & Hearing Disorders* 39, pp379–94.

Bloodstein O, 1995, *A Handbook on Stuttering*, 5th Edition, Singular, San Diego, CA.

Botterill W, Kelman E & Rustin L, 1991, 'Parents and their pre-school stuttering child', Rustin L (ed), *Parents, Families and the Stuttering Child*, Far Communications, Kibworth.

Brandes D & Phillips H, 1978, *Gamesters' Handbook*, Hutchinson, London.

British Stuttering Association, 2000, *Teenagers and Young Adults Who Stutter* (leaflet), British Stuttering Association, London.

Byrne R, 1991, *Let's Talk about Stammering*, The British Stammering Association, London.

Conture EG, 1989, *Stuttering and Your Child: Questions and Answers*, Publication No 22, Speech Foundation of America, Memphis, TN.

Conture EG, 1997, 'Evaluating childhood stuttering', Curlee RF & Siegel GM (eds), *Nature and Treatment of Stuttering: New Directions*, Allyn & Bacon, Boston, MA.

Conture EG, 2001, *Stuttering: Its Nature, Diagnosis, and Treatment*, Allyn & Bacon, Boston, MA.

Cooper E & Cooper CS, 1985, *Cooper Personalised Fluency Control Therapy*, DLM Teaching Resources, Leicester.

Cooper EB, 1993, 'Chronic perseverative stuttering syndrome: A helpful or harmful construct?', *American Journal of Speech-Language Pathology* 2 (3), pp11–15.

Corey G, 1991, *Theory and Practice of Counselling and Psychotherapy*, Brooks Cole Publishers, Belmont, CA.

Cossavella A & Hobbs C, 2002, *Farewell and Welcome: A Neat Finish and a Good Start*, Lucky Duck Books, UK.

Crowe TA & Walton JH, 1981, 'Teacher attitudes towards stuttering', *Journal of Fluency Disorders* 6, pp163–74.

Crowe TA, Di Lollo A & Crowe BT, 2000, *Crowe's Protocols: A Comprehensive Guide to Stuttering Assessment*, The Psychological Corporation, San Antonio, TX.

Curlee R, 1999, *Stuttering and Related Disorders of Fluency*, 2nd edn, Thieme, New York, NY.

Curlee R & Yairi E, 1998, 'Treatment of early childhood stuttering: Advances and research needs', *American Journal of Speech-Language Pathology* 7 (3), pp20–26.

Davis S, Howell P & Cooke F, 2002, 'Sociodynamic relationships between children who stammer and their non-stuttering classmates', *Journal of Child Psychology and Psychiatry* 43 (7), pp939–47.

De Nil LF & Brutten GJ, 1991, 'Speech-associated attitudes of stuttering and nonstuttering children', *Journal of Speech &Hearing Research* 34, pp60–66.

de Shazer S, 1991, *Putting Difference to Work*, Norton, New York, NY.

Franck AL, Jackson RA, Pimentel J & Greenwood GS, 2003, 'School-age children's perceptions of a person who stutters', *Journal of Fluency Disorders*, 28, pp1–5.

Fraser J & Perkins WH, 2000, *Do You Stutter: A Guide for Teens*, 3rd edn, Speech Foundation of America, Memphis, TN.

Gottwald SR, 1999, 'Family communication patterns and stuttering development: an analysis of the research literature', Bernstein-Ratner N & Healey EC (eds), *Stuttering Research and Practice: Bridging the Gap*, Lawrence Erlbaum Associates, Mahwah, NJ.

Gottwald SR & Hall NE, 2003, 'Stuttering treatment in schools: Developing family and teacher partnerships', *Seminars in Speech and Language* 24 (1), pp41–46.

Grove-Stevenson I & Quillam S, 1986, *Goal!*, Jonquil Publishing, Stevenage, Herts.

Gustafson M, 1996, *Snooky the Snail's Preschool Worksheets*, Super Duper School Company, Greenville, SC.

Hall FH, 2000, 'Framework for multicultural considerations in the assessment and treatment of stuttering', Baker KL, Rustin L & Cook F (eds), *Proceedings of the Fifth Oxford Dysfluency Conference.*

Hayhow R, 1992, 'Childhood Dysfluency': Presentation to Special Interest Group, Disorders of Fluency Study Day, Gloucester.

Hayhow R & Levy C, 1989, *Working with Stuttering*, Winslow Press, Bicester, Oxon.

Heinze BA & Johnson KL, 1987, *Easy Does It: Activities for School Aged Stutterers*, LinguiSystems Inc, Moline, IL.

Hill D, 1999, 'Evaluation of child factors related to early stuttering: A descriptive study', Bernstein-Ratner N & Healey C (eds), *Stuttering research and practice: Bridging the gap*, Lawrence Erlbaum, London.

Hill DG, 1995, 'Assessing the language of children who stutter', *Topics in Language Disorder,* 15 (3), 60–79.

Holmes TH & Masuda M, 1974, 'Life change and illness susceptibility', Dohrenwend BS & Dohrenwend BP (eds), *Stressful Life Events: Their Nature and Effects*, Wiley-Interscience, New York, NY.

Horsley IA & Fitzgibbon CT, 1987, 'Stuttering children: Investigation of a stereotype', *British Journal of Disorders of Communication* 22, pp19–35.

Hubbard C & Yairi E, 1988, 'Clustering of dysfluencies in the speech of stuttering and nonstuttering preschool children', *Journal of Speech & Hearing Research* 31, pp228–33.

Hughes C, 2003, 'Bullying – what people are telling us', *Speaking Out*, Summer, pp11–12.

Hughes C, 2003, 'Bullying – some strategies used in schools', *Speaking Out*, Winter, pp8–9.

Jackson SR, 1988, 'Self characterization: Dimensions of meaning', Fransella F & Thomas L (eds), *Experimenting with Personal Construct Psychology*, Routledge & Kegan Paul, London.

Johnson W, 1942, 'A study of the onset and development of stuttering', *Journal of Speech Disorders* 7, pp251–57.

Johnson W, 1946, *People in Quandaries*, Harper Brothers, New York, NY.

Johnson W, 1955, 'The time, the place and the problem', Johnson W & Leutenegger RR (eds), *Stuttering in Children and Adults*, University of Minnesota Press, Minneapolis, MN.

Johnson W, 1959, *The Onset of Stuttering*, University of Minnesota Press, Minneapolis, MN.

Kelly EM & Conture EG, 1992, 'Speaking rates, response time latencies, and interrupting behaviours of young stutterers, nonstutterers, and their mothers', *Journal of Speech and Hearing Research* 35, pp1256–67.

Kelly GA, 1991, *The Psychology of Personal Constructs*, Routledge, London.

Lass NJ, Ruscello DM, Schmitt JF, Paanbacker MD, Orlando MB, Dean KA, Ruziska JC & Bradshaw KH, 1992, 'Teachers' perceptions of stutterers', *Language, Speech and Hearing Services in Schools* 23, pp78–81.

Lees R & Boyle B, 1993, *Clinical teaching in an intensive therapy course for adults who stutter*, paper presented at Special Interest Group (dysfluency) study day, Glasgow.

Levy C, 1987, 'Interiorised stuttering: A group therapy approach', Levy C (ed), *Stuttering Therapies: Practical Approaches*, Croom Helm, London.

Madders J, 1987, *Relax and Be Happy*, Unwin, London.

Manning WH, 2001, *Clinical Decision Making in Fluency Disorders*, Singular, Memphis, TN.

Markham U, 1990, *Helping Children Cope with Stress*, Sheldon Press, London.

McGough R & Rosen M, 1981, *You Tell Me!*, Puffin, London.

McNeil C, Thomas C, Maggs B & Taylor S, 2003, *The Swindon Fluency Packs*, Swindon Primary Care Trust, Swindon.

Myers SC & Woodford LL, 1992, *The Fluency Development System*, United Educational Services, Buffalo, NY.

Nightingale C, 1986, *Who am I?*, Jonquil Publishing, Stevenage, Herts.

Onslow M & Packman A, 1999, 'The Lidcombe program of early stuttering intervention', Bernstein-Ratner N & Healey C (eds), *Stuttering Research & Practice*, Lawrence Erlbaum Associates, London, New Jersey.

Oyler E & Ramig P, 1995, *Vulnerability in stuttering children*, mini-seminar presented at the annual American Speech & Language Hearing Convention, Orlando, FL.

Packman A & Onslow M, 2000, 'The Lidcombe program for early stuttering: The old and the new', *Proceedings of the Third World Congress of Fluency*, Nyborg, Denmark.

Palomares S & Schilling D, 2001, *How to Handle a Bully*, Innerchoice, Torrance, CA.

Peters TJ & Guitar B, 1991, *Stuttering: An integrated approach to its nature and treatment*, Williams and Wilkins, Baltimore, MD.

Perkins W, 1992, *Stuttering Prevented*, Singular Publishing Company Inc, San Diego, CA.

Ravenette AT, 1977, 'Psychological investigation of children and young people', Bannister D (ed), *New Perspectives in Personal Construct Theory*, Academic Press, London.

Ravenette AT, 1980, 'The exploration of consciousness: Personal construct intervention with children', Landfield A & Leitner L (eds), *Personal Construct Psychology: Psychotherapy and Personality*, John Wiley & Sons, New York, NY.

Reid T, 1987, 'Intensive block modification therapy', Levy C (ed), *Stuttering Therapies: Practical Approaches*, Croom Helm, London.

Rickard J, 1996, *Relaxation for Children*, Acer, Melbourne.

Riley G & Riley J, 1983, 'Evaluation as a basis for intervention', Prins D & Ingham R (eds), *Treatment of stuttering in early childhood: Methods and issues*, Singular, San Diego, CA.

Riley GD, 1994, *Stuttering Severity Instrument for Children and Adults*, 3rd edn, Pro-Ed, Austin, TX.

Rogers CR, 1957, 'The necessary and sufficient conditions of therapeutic personality change', *Journal of Consulting Psychology* 21, pp95–123.

Rustin L, 1987, *Assessment and Therapy Programme for Dysfluent Children*, NFER Publishing Company Ltd, Windsor, Berks.

Rustin L & Kuhr A, 1989, *Social Skills and the Speech Impaired*, Taylor & Francis, London.

Rustin L & Purser H, 1991, 'Child development, families and the problem of stuttering', Rustin L (ed), *Parents, Families and the Stuttering Child*, Far Communications, Kibworth.

Rustin L, Botterill W & Cook F, 1991, 'Intensive management of the adolescent stutterer', Rustin L (ed), *Parents, Families and the Stuttering Child*, Far Communications, Kibworth.

Rustin L, Spence R & Cook F, 1994, 'The communication skills approach: Management of stuttering in adolescence', *First World Congress on Fluency Disorders Proceedings*, Vol 11, Munich,

Rustin L, Spence R & Cook F, 1995, *Management of Stuttering in Adolescence: A Communication Skills Approach*, Whurr Publishers Ltd, London.

Rustin L, Cook F, Botterill W, Hughes C & Kelman E, 2001, *Stammering: A Practical Guide for Teachers and other Professionals*, David Fulton, London.

Ryan BP, 1992, 'Articulation, language, rate, and fluency characteristics of stuttering and non stuttering preschool children', *Journal of Speech and Hearing Research* 35, pp333–42.

Shapiro DA, 1999, *Stuttering Intervention*, Pro-Ed Inc, Austin, TX.

Sheehan JG, 1958, 'Conflict theory of stuttering', Eisenson J (ed), *Stuttering: A Symposium*, Harper & Row, New York, NY.

Sheehan JG, 1970, *Stuttering: Research & Therapy*, Harper & Row, New York, NY.

Sheehan JG, 1975, 'Conflict theory and avoidance reduction therapy', Eisenson J (ed), *Stuttering: A Second Symposium*, Harper & Row, New York, NY.

Sheehan JG & Martyn MM, 1966, 'Spontaneous recovery from stuttering', *Journal of Speech & Hearing Research 9*, pp121–135.

Smith G, 2002, 'Freeing the self: Using psychodrama techniques with children and adolescents who stammer', Bannister A & Huntington A (eds), *Communicating with Children and Adolescents: Action for Change*, Jessica Kingsley, London.

Starkweather CW, 1981, 'Speech fluency and its development in normal children', Lass N (ed), *Speech and Language: Advances in Basic Research and Practice*, vol 4, Academic Press, New York, NY.

Starkweather CW, 1985, 'The development of fluency in normal children', *Stuttering Therapy: Prevention and Intervention with Children*, Speech Foundation of America, Memphis, TN.

Starkweather CW, 1987, *Fluency and Stuttering*, Prentice Hall, Englewood Cliffs, NJ.

Starkweather CW, 1999, 'The effectiveness of stuttering therapy: An issue for science?', Bernstein-Ratner N & Healey EC (eds), *Stuttering Research and Practice: Bridging the Gap*, Lawrence Erlbaum, London.

Starkweather CW & Gottwald SR, 1990, 'The demands and capacities model 11: Clinical applications', *Journal of Fluency Disorders* 15, pp143–57.

Stewart T & Turnbull J, 1995, *Working with Dysfluent Children*, 1st edn, Winslow Press, Bicester, Oxon.

Stones R, 1993, *Don't Pick On Me: How to Handle Bullying*, Piccadilly Press, London.

Sunderland M & Engleheart P, 1993, *Draw on your Emotions*, Winslow Press, Bicester, Oxon.

Susca M & Healy EC, 2000, 'Multifactorial Issues in the Assessment of Stuttering', *Journal of Fluency Disorders* 25 (3), pp213–18.

Thompson D, Arora T & Sharp S, 2002, *Bullying: Effective Strategies for Long Term Improvement*, Routledge Falmer, London.

Throneberg R & Yairi E, 2001, 'Durational, proportionate and absolute frequency characteristics of dysfluencies: A longitudinal study regarding persistence and recovery', *Journal of Speech, Language & Hearing Research* 44, pp38–51.

Throneberg RN & Yairi E, 1994, 'Temporal dynamics of repetitions during the early stage of childhood stuttering', *Journal of Speech and Hearing Research* 37, pp1067–75.

Turnbull J & Stewart T, 1996, *Helping Children Cope with Stammering*, Sheldon Press, London.

Turnbull J & Stewart T, 1999, *The Dysfluency Resource Book*, Winslow Press, Bicester, Oxon.

Turner JS & Helms DB, 1991, *Lifespan Development*, Holt, Rinehart & Winston, Fort Worth, TX.

Van Riper C, 1973, *The Treatment of Stuttering*, Prentice Hall, Englewood Cliffs, NJ.

Van Riper C, 1982, *The Nature of Stuttering*, Prentice Hall, Englewood Cliffs, NJ.

Van Riper C, 1987, 'A personal message', Fraser J & Perkins WH (eds), *Do you Stutter? A Guide for Teenagers*, Speech Foundation of America, Memphis, TN.

Van Riper C, 1990, 'Final thoughts about stuttering', *Journal of Fluency Disorders* 15, pp317–18.

Varnava G, 2003, *How to stop bullying in your school: A guide for teachers*, David Fulton, London.

Watkins RV & Yairi E, 1997, 'Language production abilities of children whose stuttering persisted or recovered', *Journal of Speech, Language and Hearing Research* 40, pp385–99.

Watzlawick P, Weakland J & Fisch R, 1974, *Change: Principles of Problem Formulation and Problem Resolution*, Norton, New York, NY.

Waugh MG, 1991, *Winning in Speech*, The Speech Bin, Norcross. GA.

Whitaker DS & Lieberman MA, 1964, *Psychotherapy through the Group Process*, Aldine, NY.

Williams DE, 1987, 'Coping with Parents', Fraser J & Perkins WH (eds), *Do you stutter: A Guide for Teens*, Speech Foundation of America, Memphis, TN.

Williams R & Whitehead S, 2000, 'Lidcombe therapy at the compass centre for clinical education and therapy', City University, *Lidcombe News* 13.

Wilson P, 1988, *Games Without Frontiers*, Marshall Pickering, London.

Woods CL, 1974, 'Social position and speaking competence of stuttering and normally fluent males', *Journal of Speech & Hearing Research* 17, pp740–47.

Woods S, Shearsby J, Onslow M & Burnham D, 2002, 'Psychological impact of the Lidcombe program of early stuttering intervention', *International Journal of Language & Communication Disorders* 37, 1, pp31–40.

Wright L & Ayre A, 2000, *WASSP: The Wright & Ayre Stuttering Self-Rating Profile* Speechmark, Bicester, Oxon.

Yairi E, 1983, 'The onset of stuttering in 2- and 3-year-old children: A preliminary report', *Journal of Speech & Hearing Research* 24, pp490–95.

Yairi E, 1997, 'Disfluencies of normally speaking two-year-old children', *Journal of Speech and Hearing Research* 24, pp490–95.

Yairi E, 1997, 'Disfluency characteristics of childhood dysfluency', Curlee RF & Siegel GM (eds), *Nature and Treatment of Stuttering: New Directions*, 2nd edn, Allyn & Bacon, Boston, MA.

Yairi E, 2000, 'The Changing Models of Stuttering Development: Research Findings and Clinical Implications', Baker KL, Rustin L & Cook F (eds), *Proceedings of the Fifth Oxford Dysfluency Conference*, Oxford.

Yairi E & Ambrose N, 1992, 'A longitudinal study of stuttering children: A preliminary report', *Journal of Speech & Hearing Research* 35, pp755–60.

Yairi, E & Ambrose N, 1992, 'Onset of stuttering in preschool children: Selected factors', *Journal of Speech & Hearing Research* 35, pp782–88.

Yairi E & Ambrose N, 1999, 'Early childhood stuttering 1: Persistency and recovery rates', *Journal of Speech, Language & Hearing Research* 42, pp1097–112.

Yairi E & Lewis B, 1984, 'Disfluencies at the Onset of Stuttering', *Journal of Speech and Hearing Research* 27, 154–59.

Yairi E, Ambrose N & Niermann R, 1993, 'The early months of stuttering: A developmental study', *Journal of Speech & Hearing Research* 36, pp521–28.

Yairi E, Ambrose N, Paden E & Throneberg R, 1996, 'Predictive factors of persistence and recovery: Pathways of childhood stuttering', *Journal of Communication Disorders* 29, 51–77.

Yalom ID, 1985, *The Theory and Practice of Group Psychotherapy*, Basic Books, New York, NY.

Yaruss S, 2004, 'Documenting individual treatment outcomes in stuttering therapy', *Contemporary Issues in Communication Science and Disorders* 31, Dec, pp49–57.

Yaruss S, 2005, 'Measuring multiple outcomes in stuttering treatment', *Proceedings of the Sixth Oxford Dysfluency Conference*, Oxford.

Yaruss S & Reeves L, 2002, *Pioneering stuttering research in the 21st century: the first joint symposium for scientists and consumers: Summary report and proceedings*, National Stuttering Association, Anaheim, CA.

Yeakle MK & Cooper EB, 1986, 'Teacher Perceptions of Stuttering', *Journal of Fluency Disorders* 11, pp345–59.

Yovetich WMS, Leschied AW & Flicht J, 2000, 'Self-esteem of school-age children who stutter', *Journal of Fluency Disorders* 25, pp143–53.

Zebrowski PM, 1995, 'The Topography of Beginning Stuttering' *Journal of Communication Disorders* 28, pp75–91.

Index

construing of dysfluency 85
group therapy 162, 186–7
intervention 86–95
length of time apparent 85
and normal non-fluency 85
parents 86–95
recovery from stammering 49–53
repetitions 49, 53, 255
schools 231
working with the child 95–7
easy onset 120–3
embarrassment 6, 135, 145, 261
emotions/feelings 30–1, 75, 78, 141, 207–8, 261
demands on child 39–40
negative 39, 88, 143–6
parents 88–9
recognition 111, 140
empowering children 269, 270–1
empowering parents 89, 271
Engleheart P 75
environment 87, 93–4
change 92–3
demands of 34, 36–8, 59
fluency disrupters 90–2
and speech 36–7
events, demands of 13–14, 39
expectations of child 7
experts: non-expert stance 18–19
eye contact 16, 62, 110
group therapy 202–3

F
facial expression 110–11
facts about stammering 249, 263, 264
family
see also parents
attitudes to speech 7–9
attitudes to stammering 94
avoidance behaviour 272
and borderline stammering 107–8
busyness 12
and change 107–8
communication 5, 9–12, 90, 156, 191, 271
discipline 12
expectations of child 7
in group therapy 173–4
history 6
interaction 11, 38, 93–4
lifestyle 94

partnership with clinicians and teachers 231
family trees 140, 215
famous people who stammer 263, 265
Farewell and Welcome (Cossavella & Hobbs) 244
feedback
from parents 129
group therapy 178, 217
feelings *see* emotions/feelings
fluency
attitudes of peer group 107
basal levels of 95
control 209–10
disrupters 15–16, 41, 90–2, 95–6
focusing on 129
and non-fluency 2, 129, 250
strategies 271–2
fluency disrupters 15–16, 90–2
focusing on non-fluency 129, 250
follow-up in group therapy 163
'Fraidy the cat' (Waugh) 209
Franck AL 220–1
frequency of dysfluencies 51, 67–8
friendships
borderline stammering 102, 104–6
boys and girls 105–6
in schools 226
and teasing/bullying 238, 240

G
games
group therapy 217–18
teacher training sessions 256–7
gelling: group therapy 187–8, 204
gender 51, 52, 60, 262, 263
genetic factors in stammering 46, 60, 262, 263
genograms 140, 215
gestures 111–12
Gottwald SR 30, 88–9, 93–4, 220, 231
group therapy 160–81, 185–218
accommodation 163, 166–7
advantages 160–1, 211
aims 164, 167
borderline stammering 192–3
confirmed stammering 211–12
for parents of younger children 186
attendance 166
borderline stammering 162, 192–3, 192–211

teacher training 248

R

Ramig P 30
Ravenette AT 139–40
reactions to stammering *see* attitudes to
    stammering
reading aloud 104, 153–4, 235
reconstruing stammering 102, 143–4
    confirmed stammering 142–6
    and peer group 106
recording: group therapy 177–9
recordings (video/audio) 64–5, 90
recovery from stammering 84, 87
    early dysfluency 49–53
    and persistence 51–3
Reeves L 268
registration, school 104, 224, 226, 234
relaxation techniques 127–8, 199
religious events and stress 13
repertory grids 138
repetitions 66
    borderline stammering 100, 255
    development of stammering 49, 53, 60
    early dysfluency 49, 53, 255
reports: group therapy 179
research on stammering 24–5
respiration 120, 128, 200
rhythm, sense of 29–30
Rickard J 127
Riley G & J 30
Riley GD 67, 68, 70
risk factors 87
Rogers CR 11
role reversal 141
role-playing 111–12, 113
    bullying 149
    clinicians and 208
    group therapy
        borderline stammering 199, 201
        confirmed stammering 149, 215–16
    teacher training sessions 254
roles 172–7
    and commonality 218
Royal College of Speech and Language
    Therapists 62
Rustin L 63, 151–2, 156, 207, 209
Ryan BP 71

S

SATs 225
scaling 75
Schilling D 151
schools 104, 220–66
    avoidance behaviour 230
    borderline stammering 108, 231
    classroom organisation 223–5
    confirmed stammering 137, 145, 231
    conspiracy of silence 228
    construing dysfluency 227, 228, 230–1
    developing strategies 230–3
    discussion with teachers 175, 227–9
    early dysfluency 231
    information provided 231–2
    information shared 232–3
    liaison visits 242–5
    observation 223–6
    preparation for secondary school
        242–5
    presentations on stammering 260–6
        information 262–5
        story 265–6
    problem areas 234–6
    studies 220–1
    teacher's perspective 272
    teasing and bullying 233, 237–42
    visiting 222–42
sculpting group therapy 216–17
secondary symptoms 69–70, 85
self, view of 102, 103, 106, 138–9, 142–3
self-esteem 31, 139, 273, 274
self-rating scales (assessment) 81
semantics, development of 35
sensitivity 30
severity of stammering 69
sex of children in group therapy 194, 213
Shapiro DA 68, 69, 70–1, 72–3, 156
Sheehan J 25, 31, 46
    icebergs 74, 189, 191, 232, 248, 254
siblings 173
    reaction to stammering 9–10
situations 139, 272
    avoidance of 134, 135–6
    difficult 272
    reconstruing 144
skills, development of 31–2, 33
SLDs (Stammer-like dysfluencies) 50, 51,
    52, 60, 66
Smith, G 141
smooth and bumpy speech 76, 123, 198–9